"James Houston and Michael Parker have written an outstanding book which is practical and rich with resources. Their knowledge of the aging process is exceptional. I heartily endorse *A Vision for the Aging Christian* as must-reading for all grandparents!"

—KEN CANFIELD,
founder, National Association for Grandparenting

"This book is built on research and scientific knowledge but goes well beyond that structure. It offers transparent examples from the authors' lives, real life examples from the lives of others, pungent quotes from well-known authors, and resources to help those caring for the aged. This is a gem, so I encourage you not to miss out on this one."

—JUDD SWIHART,
director, Cornerstone Family Counseling Center

"What a gift! James Houston and Michael Parker have given readers a clear, comprehensive, and thoughtful text addressing critical aspects of the aging process—all through the lens of Christian values. Their work provides the reader easily understood information as well as access to important resources to support successful aging. I recommend *A Vision for the Aging Christian* as a resource for individuals, families, as well as professionals in the medical and human services fields."

—JAMES MARTIN,
professor emeritus of social work and social research, Bryn Mawr College

"My friends and mentors, James Houston and Michael Parker, continue to write collaboratively and share their wisdom and passion to advocate and offer resources for elders, care partners, faith organizations, and the community at large to create a culture in which elders may go on living well. They comprehensively address issues associated with aging, offering well-researched insights and rich, illustrative stories to further a culture of compassion, dignity, and fruitfulness in elderhood. You will want to come back to this book again and again to inform and inspire."

—DANIEL C. POTTS,
neurologist

"This new book by James Houston and Michael Parker shares their double expertise in the needy field of aging Christians and their caregivers. The chapters are full of rich personal experiences and stories that inform, challenge, and encourage the reader. This whole collection which the James Houston Center for Aging has gathered together in one volume is a treasure to be explored, enjoyed, and applied."

—KAY BASCOM,
author of *Jubilee Journey: Hope from Now to Eternity*

"I believe *A Vision for the Aging Christian* will serve as a call to awaken the church to rise up and care for the aging segment of the church worldwide. This book is not an academic book but rather a practical 'hands on' guide to encourage believers and churches everywhere to meet the needs of the exploding percentage of aging people around us and throughout our world. Every page is wonderfully insightful."

—HAL HABECKER,
founder and president, Finishing Well Ministries

"The book's spiritual wisdom, the personal honesty of the authors, the up-to-date research on aging, and the critique of ageism in both the culture at large and in the church make this a very important work. I have found it encouraging and challenging both personally and clinically and recommend it wholeheartedly regardless of one's vocation or place in life."

—STEPHEN F. VOORHIES,
physician

"The authors have succeeded in giving guidance to all individuals who are interested in living wisely with purpose and resilience despite whatever challenges they face. They have focused on the challenges associated with aging. They share personal faith journeys and provide evidence-based guidance that have great practical applications. Inclusion of specific guidance on developing a parent care readiness plan and conducting life reviews make this book an especially helpful and unique resource."

—RICHARD M. ALLMAN,
clinical professor of medicine, George Washington University

A Vision for the Aging Christian

A Vision for the Aging Christian

Preparing for Longer Life and the Tasks of Caregiving

JAMES M. HOUSTON & MICHAEL PARKER

CASCADE *Books* · Eugene, Oregon

A VISION FOR THE AGING CHRISTIAN
Preparing for Longer Life and the Tasks of Caregiving

Copyright © 2024 James M. Houston and Michael Parker. All rights reserved. Except for brief quotations in critical publications or reviews, no part of this book may be reproduced in any manner without prior written permission from the publisher. Write: Permissions, Wipf and Stock Publishers, 199 W. 8th Ave., Suite 3, Eugene, OR 97401.

Cascade Books
An Imprint of Wipf and Stock Publishers
199 W. 8th Ave., Suite 3
Eugene, OR 97401

www.wipfandstock.com

PAPERBACK ISBN: 978-1-6667-4120-9
HARDCOVER ISBN: 978-1-6667-4121-6
EBOOK ISBN: 978-1-6667-4122-3

Cataloguing-in-Publication data:

Names: Houston, James M. | Parker, Michael

Title: A Vision for the Aging Christian : Preparing for Longer Life and the Tasks of Caregiving / James M. Houston and Michael Parker.

Description: Eugene, OR: Cascade Books, 2024 | Includes bibliographical references and index.

Identifiers: ISBN 978-1-6667-4120-9 (paperback) | ISBN 978-1-6667-4121-6 (hardcover) | ISBN 978-1-6667-4122-3 (ebook)

Subjects: LCSH: Older people—Conduct of life. | Aging—Religious aspects—Christianity. | Aging—Social aspects.

Classification: HQ1061 V54159 2024 (paperback) | HQ1061(ebook)

10/29/24

Scripture quotations marked CEV are from the Contemporary English Version Copyright © 1995 by American Bible Society. Used by permission. All rights reserved.

Scripture quotations marked CSB are from the Christian Standard Bible. Copyright © 2017 by Holman Bible Publishers. Used by permission. Christian Standard Bible® and CSB® are federally registered trademarks of Holman Bible Publishers, all rights reserved.

Scripture quotations marked ESV are from The Holy Bible, English Standard Version. Copyright © 2001 by Crossway Bibles, a publishing ministry of Good News

Publishers. Used by permission. All rights reserved.

Scripture quotations marked KJ21 are from the 21st Century King James Version. Copyright © 1994 by Deuel Enterprises, Inc. Used by permission. All rights reserved.

Scripture quotations marked MSG are from The Message. Copyright © 2018 by Eugene H. Peterson. Used by permission. All rights reserved.

Scripture quotations marked NASB® 1995 are from the New American Standard Bible®, copyright © 1995 by The Lockman Foundation. Used by permission. All rights reserved. lockman.org.

Scripture quotations marked NASB® 2020 are from the New American Standard Bible®, copyright © 2020 by The Lockman Foundation. Used by permission. All rights reserved. lockman.org.

Scripture quotations marked NIV® are from the New International Version®, copyright © 2011 by Biblica, Inc.® Used by permission. All rights reserved worldwide.

Scripture quotations marked NKJV are from the New King James Version®. Copyright © 1982 by Thomas Nelson. Used by permission. All rights reserved.

Scripture quotations marked NRSVA are from the New Revised Standard Version Bible: Anglicised Catholic Edition, copyright © 1995 the Division of Christian Education of the National Council of the Churches of Christ in the United States of America. Used by permission. All rights reserved.

Scripture quotations marked NRSVUE are from the New Revised Standard Version, Updated Edition. Copyright © 2021 National Council of Churches of Christ in the United States of America. Used by permission. All rights reserved worldwide.

Scripture quotations marked RSV are from the Revised Standard Version of the Bible, 2nd ed., copyright © 1971 by the Division of Christian Education of the National Council of the Churches of Christ in the United States of America. Used by permission. All rights reserved.

Contents

Foreword by Michael Parker | *xiii*

Prologue | *xv*

I. OUR STORIES OF FAITH

CHAPTER 1
Introduction | 3

CHAPTER 2
Dr. Houston's Stories of God's Providence, Favor, and Purpose | 16

CHAPTER 3
Mike's Stories of God's Providence, Favor, and Purpose | 18

II. OUR SPIRITUAL-EMOTIONAL SIDE

CHAPTER 4
Prayer as Friendship with God | 27

CHAPTER 5
Learning to Dwell in His Presence: Places of Prayer | 32

CHAPTER 6
Maturing in Holiness | 45

CHAPTER 7
A Respite in the Storm: A Place for Miracles | 53

CHAPTER 8
Life Review: Leaving an Intergenerational Legacy | 60

III. OUR AGING MINDS

CHAPTER 9
Sleep | 79

CHAPTER 10
Facing the Epidemic of Dementia: A Present-Day Leprosy? | 85

IV. OUR SELVES IN COMMUNITY

CHAPTER 11
A Christian's Caregiving Ministry | 107

CHAPTER 12
Caregiving for Aging Parents and Loved Ones | 110

CHAPTER 13
AgeReady | 124

CHAPTER 14
The Gift of Blessing the Next Generation | 137

Epilogue: Jim Houston's Farewell Letter Written on the Eve of His Hundredth Birthday | 139

Appendices: Faith-Based Programs | 147

    Appendix A: Introduction | 149

    Appendix B: Faith-Based Initiatives in Support of America's Veterans | 152

    Appendix C: The Eric Liddell Community of Today | 155

    Appendix D: A Short History of the Eric Liddell Centre/Community | 157

    Appendix E: Cognitive Dynamics | 165

    Appendix F: Finishing Well Ministries | 167

    Appendix G: Spreading the Model of Dementia-Focused Respite Ministry | 169

    Appendix H: Grandparents Matter: Supporting Grandparenting | 171

Appendix I: Faith in Older People | 173

Appendix J: Tuscaloosa Senior Ministry Projects | 175

Appendix K: Small Volunteer Ministries That Can Bless Older People | 178

Appendix L: Senior Ministry Associations | 180

Bibliography | 183

Biographies | 194

Index | 195

Foreword

THIS BOOK MELDS THE WISDOM of Dr. James Houston, a one-hundred-year-old internationally renowned theologian, with the expertise and research of a noted Christian gerontologist. Its primary aims are to help the aging Christian prepare for her or his last season of life with purpose, resiliency, and faithfulness; and to address specific areas of challenge for the church of aging persons and their caregivers. Alzheimer's disease spares no one its suffering, yet we offer a fresh look at this problem. It includes substantial reviews of dementia, family caregiving, and an introduction of the AgeReady Program, which includes the tasks of caregiving, and detailed reviews on years of caregiving research with varied groups: military families, university faculties, and congregations. It discusses scientifically based information about dementia and caregiving, and vignettes and anecdotes drawn from the lives and careers of Drs. Houston and Parker and their colleagues. A focus is on faithful, purposeful, Christian living in the face of chronic disease and dementia. It will be of use to individual Christians seeking to make the most of their later years, and to congregations in their work with and for older adults and their caregivers. It contains appendices that hold synoptic descriptions by leaders of other greatly needed, Christian, age-friendly programs, and connections with these leaders and access to their resources. We are committed to helping the reader to think creatively by thinking globally and acting locally. We are using new technologies for Christian leaders to share in developing aging veteran programs, age-friendly, dementia respite programs for family caregivers, life review programs, faith and successful aging conferences, senior ministry associations, grandparent support programs, Finishing Well Ministries, nursing home visitation programs, and more.

Prologue

I REMEMBER OUR FIRST community-based faith and successful aging conference over twenty-five years ago. Many of the organizers are dead, as are some of the presenters. As I looked the seniors in attendance square in the eye and declared, "We need you today! Your grandchildren need you! Your heavenly Father has purpose for you!," I could see the tears of several older saints on the front row. I assumed at that time that I had struck a spiritual chord. Now we have a center with over fifty of the world's proven leaders in the many disciples from the field of aging working with us to make an age-friendly difference in the lives of our elders. As stated before, in our first book, we want to "raise up an army of senior saints, who aim to turn the world upside down for good with the love of Christ!"[1] Before we focus on the individual aging Christian and the important topics like caregiving and dementia, we need to start with some basic themes of aging that Harold Koenig of Duke School of Medicine and I covered with the special editor of *Psychology Today*.[2]

Contrary to popular opinion, aging does not begin at sixty-five. Though we may be less conscious of aging in our younger years, the truth is that from birth on we are all aging. Aging refers to the chronological, biological, psychological, social, and spiritual aspects of life over time. In a broad sense aging refers to changes that occur in the person throughout his/her life course. As we age, we move through a number of stages, typically affected by societal expectations. All societies are age graded in the sense that we are given different roles, opportunities, and status based on our age. Now that people are living longer, there is a growing interest in

---

1. Houston and Parker, *Vision for Aging Church*, 22.
2. Aten, "Aging with Resilience."

understanding the process of aging, which has resulted in increasing interest in the multidisciplinary fields of gerontology.

Gerontologists study the biological, psychological, social, and spiritual aspects of aging. There are multiple theories about how we age, from the description of cellular processes associated with aging to the study of how we define successful aging. It is important to make a distinction between gerontology, which takes a cradle-to-grave perspective, and geriatrics, which is the medical treatment of older persons. Most experts would agree that avoiding disease and disability, maximizing cognitive and physical fitness, being actively engaged in life, and growing in our level of spiritual and emotional maturity are key aspects of "successful" aging. More recently, terms like "optimal aging" are increasingly being used in order to capture the fact that not everyone is able to achieve successful aging as we defined it previously.[3] For some, perhaps most of us, we'll need to learn how to grow in our faith as we learn to accept help in some areas of life. In this book we hope to focus on how persons navigate their limited personal, economic, and social resources to solve problems (exhibit problem-solving, self-efficacy, and self-reliance), while growing in spiritual maturity and capacity to love and care for others. Much of our research at the center has addressed the spiritual aspects of life, health, and aging, including elder caregiving and proactive planning for those are seeking to learn more about to live longer lives of purpose.

Given the healthy response to our first book, *A Vision for the Aging Church*,[4] we have been careful to provide a better system for responding to age-friendly questions about best practices for living life as unique human beings. We have named our center the Center for Faith and Successful Aging in honor of this book's coauthor, Scottish-born Dr. James Houston.[5] At one hundred plus, Jim embodies the successful aging senior with a purpose-driven, spiritually mature life. It is not that Jim has not faced health challenges like most older people. It is his capacity to stay on track with his God-given purposes that is noteworthy, and that he remains creatively resilient in harmony with his centenarian status. His late-life accomplishments include the sharing of lessons he learned from his extensive caregiving duties with his wife, Rita, after she was diagnosed with Alzheimer's disease.

3. Crowther et al., "Rowe and Kahn's Model."
4. Houston and Parker, *Vision for Aging Church*.
5. See www.jameshoustoncenter.com.

PROLOGUE

In his ninety-eighth and ninety-ninth years, Jim ran a weekly Zoom Bible study with over twenty Christians participating from all over the US, which was quickly followed by weekly emails to hundreds of followers who had signed up for regular doses of his wisdom and biblical perspective. The world is packed full of "experts," but few have reached the age of one hundred. He has been and will continue to be a source of wisdom through his written work for all who have the courage to admit that they are aging. It is my honor and responsibility, as a witness, to help capture some snapshots of his journey and mine that may prove helpful to you in your own journey as a lifelong learner and disciple of Christ.

Wisdom is not something that can be proven by argument or debate. Wisdom must meet the test of time.[6] Jim's story of being freed by God's grace from childhood insecurity helped him live a life of boldness "in Christ." Many are the growing number of disciples of Jesus who have looked to Jim as a "spiritual father." He speaks in humility into our lives through his example, his lectures and teaching, and his writing. Soon, his son Christopher may publish some of the letters he wrote in 2022 that testify of Christ's love and mercy to him and others over the decades, which include his memories of his life and service during World War I.

Through our understanding of the Scriptures and the science of aging, we hope to provide a guide to aging wisely and successfully with purpose and resilience amid the challenges of this world. We aim to encourage you to live a life on the edge and show you how exciting it can be when God himself, our Creator and the King of kings, shows a personal interest in you and the plans he has for you.[7] It means that we must be truly open to God's mystical presence in the world and to his invitations to engage with the world's problems and challenges, including the pandemics and calamities of life like COVID, or chronic diseases like arthritis and the frightening dementias. We must help and provide aid to aging veterans and first responders, and to the victims of sex trafficking and natural disasters. Nor can we dodge the latest war and its unfathomable acts of racist violence against older people, infants, babies, the traumatized, the wounded, and the disabled. As we look to the future with all of these and more challenges, we pray that our Triune God will reveal and confirm his unique, late-life purposes for you. Like the old military recruitment posters, "We need you!"

---

6. Blackaby et al., *Experiencing God*.
7. Houston, *Joyful Exiles*.

I. Our Stories of Faith

Chapter 1

Introduction

But if any of you lacks wisdom, let him ask of God, who gives to all generously and without reproach, and it will be given to him. (Jas 1:5 NASB 2020)

And even when I am old and gray, God, do not abandon me, / Until I declare Your strength to this generation, Your power to all who are to come. (Ps 71:18 NASB 2020)

"And it shall be in the last days," God says, "That I will pour out My Spirit on all mankind; / And your sons and your daughters will prophesy, / And your young men will see visions, / And your old men will have dreams." (Acts 2:17 NASB 2020)

For we are His workmanship, created in Christ Jesus for good works, which God prepared beforehand so that we would walk in them. (Eph 2:10 NASB 2020)

This is what the Lord says: / "Stand by the ways and see and ask for the ancient paths, / Where the good way is, and walk in it; / Then you will find a resting place for your souls." (Jer 6:16 NASB 2020)

LOOKING BACK AT OUR EARLIER WORK AND FIRST BOOK

Just a few years ago, I (Mike) was introduced to a remarkable man, Dr. James Houston. Not only is he a tested source of wisdom at one hundred plus, but he is also an excellent example of successful aging, who has a heart for the highly neglected topic of aging. In the process of coauthoring our first book, *A Vision for the Aging Church*, I happily discovered that Jim adheres to the highly relational, tutorial style of mentoring used widely at Oxford in the 1940s and made famous as a preeminent form of education by Christian scholars like Jim's friend and colleague C. S. Lewis. Under this system the tutor and pupil often attained a level of intimacy and lifelong friendship that is rarely seen in today's top graduate schools, where academic and political correctness and artificial educational boundaries act as deterrents to most forms of genuine friendship between a professor and a student. Based upon the paideia model of education, the tutor or "don" at Oxford focused on the character and wholistic (body, mind, heart, and spirit) development of the student as future leader. And so, thankfully, I became another one of Jim's pupils, open to his wholistic style of friendship in Christ, and he became an invaluable member of my social convoy of family and friends.[1]

In our second book, *A Vision for the Aging Christian*, Jim and I hope to give the reader the same paideia-like learning experience that was used at Oxford years ago. We hope to approach this wholistically with a focus on body, soul, mind, and spirit. With the gospel as our foundation, we aim to share some of our personal stories of God's unsurpassed mercy and grace.[2]

As we write, *A Vision for the Aging Church: Renewing Ministry to and from Seniors* remains in press, is in its fifth printing, and has been translated into Chinese and other languages and formats. Since it was first published, we have learned much from our readers. We have received hundreds of messages from leaders of ministries, faith-based gerontologists, business leaders, entrepreneurs, and others, as well as requests to speak at Christian and professional conferences. We have worked with national and international Christian ministries and military chaplains for the US Air Force and Army; conducted eldercare research and training at the U.S. Air and Army War Colleges (the senior leadership schools of the Army and Air Force); helped two churches evaluate an eldercare training program; organized multiple conferences on Faith and Successful Aging to a broad range of faith-based communities; received funding for age-related research from a broad range of organizations (e.g., US Army Public Health Command, National Institute on Aging, the Hartford Foundation, Army Physical Fitness Research Institute, and others); completed a video series on spirituality and

---

1. Antonucci and Akiyama, "Convoys of Social Relations."

2. *Mercy*—God not giving us what we deserve; *Grace*—God giving us what we do not deserve.

aging for the American Association of Christian Counselors; and delivered plenary addresses to organizations like the North American Association of Christians in Social Work, Faith in Older People in Scotland, and others.

By God's grace, we hope to share highlights from some of our programs, journal articles, and peer-reviewed chapters on faith, caregiving, and successful aging.[3] These include the design and execution of the University of Alabama in Birmingham's longitudinal mobility study of one thousand seniors (five hundred white; five hundred African American; five hundred women; five hundred men). Using data from the UAB study, we completed a series of analyses that demonstrated the powerful effects of strong, vibrant faith on a variety of measures of physical and emotional health.[4] Seniors with high religious attendance and strong faith in God were among the healthiest of groups. As my now-deceased colleague and friend Dave Larson often said to me (Mike) of his research on faith and health with the National Institutes of Health and later the John Templeton Foundation, "Not surprisingly, God simply proves himself strong in all of the research we have conducted with religious and spiritual variables!"[5] Though Dave's groundbreaking work was eventually recognized by the American Psychiatric Association, he often encountered contentious colleagues, as have we, who vehemently opposed the study and measurement of anything spiritual or religious. His research essentially criticized the scientific community for neglecting to study or include "religious and spiritual" variables in their research, despite the importance of these variables in life. That mantle of leadership has shifted to Harold Koenig at Duke University, who coordinates and conducts a variety of research and teaching initiatives and archives the growing body of evidence on faith and health.[6]

Jim and I have met some remarkable elders and, most encouragingly, have seen signs of age-friendly progress by the church, faith-based organizations, Christian volunteers, and seminaries. Additionally, we have been able to come alongside some wonderful, Spirit-led directors of sustainable, local, statewide, national, and international ministries that meet genuine human needs of our elders and their family caregivers. These ministries

---

3. See, e.g., www.beageready.com.

4. Crowther et al., "Rowe and Kahn's Model."

5. Dr. Larson completed groundbreaking research that revealed the long-standing scientific bias toward the use of religious and spiritual variables in medical research across a range of disciplines.

6. See https://spiritualityandhealth.duke.edu/. Dr. Koenig serves as one of our center's partners; see www.jameshoustoncenter.com.

challenge Christian seniors to late-life purpose and leadership that make a positive difference in our ageist society. We formed the James Houston Center for Faith and Successful Aging, named in honor of Jim, which collaborates with our growing list of expert partners and seeks to promote many of their outstanding ministries in communities across the world by "thinking globally and acting locally."[7]

RESPONDING TO CRITICISM

Despite the successes of our first book, which focused on the aging church, we were challenged by colleagues and friends of our ministry to write a less academic, more personal book for aging individuals, and so we came by our title for this book together: *A Vision for the Aging Christian*. I recall a telephone conversation I had with an eighty-one-year-old, lively gentleman from Chicago, who had captured the essence of what we were trying to say in our first book: "I want to be a part of that army of senior saints you talked about in your book. I want to turn the world 'upside down' with the love of Christ too!" But he quickly added, "I didn't understand half of what you and Dr. Houston said in your first book. How do I join this army?" Not only was this dear gentleman telling us he did not understand some of what we wrote, but he was also asking for meaning and purpose to accompany his Spirit-led willingness to serve in the fields that are ripe for harvest but where the workers are few. We hear you loud and clear!

In this book, Jim and I are renewed in our commitment to translate the latest science while remaining true to sound biblical theology about aging and living with greater wisdom, purpose, and resilience. This book has been written not for theologians, but for the regular "person on the street." Much of this book contains autobiographical accounts of God's mercy, grace, and forgiveness as parts of his providential plan for our lives have unfolded. In using the genre of story, Jim and I hope to identify with other aging folk like the old "country" preacher Vernon McGee, who seemed so real, genuine, and approachable because of his attractive humility in patiently teaching the Scriptures, verse by verse.[8] When speaking at

---

7. "Thinking globally and acting locally" refers to transporting evidence-based programs from one community or agency to other communities (e.g., Faith in Older People, exporting dementia respite programs from Edinburgh to an American city or church).

8. Vernon McGee had an international radio ministry of teaching the Bible verse by verse until his death.

conferences, Reverend McGee would often say to his large audiences: "If you knew what was in my heart, you wouldn't be here; and, before you head for the exits, if I knew what was in your heart, I wouldn't be here either!" Like Reverend McGee, we want to be transparent and not neglect the joy that humor brings into the room. In writing together again, we have been inspired to claim one of Elisabeth Elliot's favorite verses that helped her cope with her first husband's martyrdom and her second husband's cancer, all the while remaining remarkably true to her vocational call as a Christian writer who touched the lives of thousands: "For the Lord God helps Me, / Therefore, I am not disgraced; / Therefore, I have made My face like flint, / And I know that I will not be ashamed. / He who vindicates Me is near" (Isa 50:7–8a NASB 2020). Jim and I are resolved to achieve the Lord's late-life purpose for ourselves. Like the autumn leaves that are nearing their end, we pray that we might bring a heavenly color to our work with you and our aging social convoy of family and friends.

CHRIST ESSENTIAL TO AGE READINESS

In this book we hope to address a broad range of topics that should be of interest to all aging people but particularly to Christian elders who aim to finish well and to become the best version of themselves in Christ. We agree with J. C. Ryle's position in *Old Paths*. Capturing the words of the prophet Jeremiah, who first used the expression "old paths" (Jer 6:16 NKJV), Ryle reassured those who followed Christ that they would find "rest for their souls." Ryle told his readers that they had no need for a new gospel. Instead, they needed the strong teaching of the "old paths." From the outset, Jim and I want to say unequivocally that we consider a relationship with Christ to be a prerequisite to aging with wisdom, resiliency, and Spirit-led purpose. As we share our stories of God's providence and favor, we hope to weave a mix of sound theology on aging with some of the latest science about how to age optimally, successfully, and faithfully. Join us then in this adventure of becoming more "age ready" personally in a world that is not typically "age friendly."

As an example of the lack of age readiness and preparedness, our published research has shown clearly that the members of three groups of committed caregivers (military families, faculty at a major university, members of congregations) are *not* prepared for the predictable, developmental challenge of caring for an aging parent, and most older people are *not* prepared for longer life and what it may bring.[9] If Jesus articulated a caregiving plan for his mother with the apostle John from the cross, how much more should we be prepared to fulfill the commandment to honor and care for our parents in late life (John 19: 26–27). Though most people have a heartfelt desire to honor their parents, they are simply "not ready" when the time comes to provide tailored, loving care. If you are an older Christian, we hope that you will take the information provided in this book to take the lead in beginning the discussions with your adult children about your long-term care plans, which should involve the completion of a series of spiritual, emotional, medical, legal-financial, and familial tasks associated with late life.

LIVING LONGER

The World Health Organization (WHO) reminds us that the number of adults aged sixty-five and above will triple from 2020 to 2050. The aging of the world's population remains a major public health issue. Our nation is already moving from a three-generational family structure to a four-tiered system, where becoming a great-grandparent is the new norm. A hundred years ago, the average person made it to the mid-thirties, while today the global life expectancy is over seventy-two and creeping upward. Despite this pattern, there is some evidence that the growing effects of chronic disease are affecting longevity in adverse ways. Nevertheless, over the next three decades, the number of sixty-year-olds will double, forcing questions for all aging persons, and Christians in particular, about what comes next. What about dementia? So many are falling victim! Both the sufferer and the caregiver . . . We plan to address these issues in some detail. If this is a journey to one hundred plus, as it has been for Jim Houston, how can we best plan and organize all those years? How do we care for our aging family and friends? Has Christ called us to care for our parents? How can we participate meaningfully in this *ageist* culture?[10] How do we navigate late-life challenges and our death-denying culture in a Christ-honoring way? Where do we turn for wise counsel? If we face chronic health conditions, are they manageable? Reversible?

---

9. Parker et al., "Parent Care and Religion."

10. *Ageism*—Prejudice or discrimination against a particular age group and especially the elderly.

INTRODUCTION

COVID-19 took a tremendous toll on all of us, but particularly on the old and disabled. Most know that our elders were particularly vulnerable and that egregious mistakes were made in the beginning days of the virus. Early in the pandemic, policymakers promulgated, for example, the placement of seniors with COVID-19 into nursing homes, which resulted in thousands of tragic, potentially avoidable deaths. One of the friends of our ministry and a great Christian leader, Joni Eareckson Tada, fought COVID-19 as a young-old person and as a quadriplegic. As we prayed for her speedy recovery, we wondered why she and other vulnerable people were not given access to the vaccine more promptly. Early research is now suggesting that those suffering from dementia who are living in long-term care facilities died at a much higher rate than other elders due to social isolation and other factors. This is one reason why we have devoted chapters to the topics of dementia and eldercare. Perhaps some of you lost a parent or grandparent to the virus without capturing their invaluable life story. Some have said that when an older saint dies, it is like burning down a library of knowledge. We have intentionally included a chapter that encourages and helps elders to tell their life stories and aids adult children in how to capture their parents' stories. This epidemic has underscored how important it is that we discuss difficult subjects proactively, while parents are able to put plans into place. We have identified almost fifty tasks that should be considered in our chapters on caregiving and the AgeReady program. In addition to the topics of caregiving and dementia, we will be covering the theological and scientific high points on a broad range of topics related to optimal, faithful, successful aging; scientifically grounded brain health strategies; iatrogenesis;[11] lifelong strategies of education, work, and respite; approaches to prayer; a theology of Christian maturity, life review, and remembrance; grandparenting; pets; widowhood; and a "good" death. Some of these topics are addressed in the AgeReady program and the appendices, which contain a treasure chest of tested, much-needed programs that can be emulated.

Our overall aim in this book is to help you enjoy God, discover his purpose for your late life, acquire his wisdom for your journey, and navigate the challenges of late life resiliently by focusing more on God and the caregiving tasks before you. And yes, we hope to raise up Christian seniors who want to turn the world upside down with the love of Christ. As we learn to focus less on ourselves and more on the needs of others and the

11. *Iatrogenesis*—Questionable, substandard medical care.

tasks of caregiving, the more we will discover an excellence in ourselves that flows from a life of faith. Thomas Merton put it this way: "A saint is not someone who is good, but who has experienced the goodness of God."[12]

As a barometer of our culture, our research confirms that many older people live under the socially sanctioned, strongly encouraged goal of retirement. Jim and I ask, "Where in the Bible does it say that Christians should retire?" Rest, yes; retire, no! Moses, Joshua, Abraham, Sarah, and others listed in the saints' hall of fame found in Heb 11 indicate that God often chooses older people for his invaluable missions. As we have noted before, most of us grew up in an antiquated, age-graded system that indicates we go to school, go to work, and then retire. We would argue that we go to school and work our entire lives, and if we are smart, we learn to take respites along the way.

Through our center's work we have learned that retirement, once achieved, can be a hollow goal for many Christians, and sometimes it can reveal a lukewarm spiritual status. We can, as Eugene Peterson has translated, choose to "run with horses" like the prophet Jeremiah did when he was metaphorically challenged by God (Jer 12:5 MSG)!

CHALLENGES OF GROWING OLDER

Geriatricians[13] use the series of *i*'s to describe many of the problems associated with late life: immobility, instability, incontinence, intellectual impairment, infection, impairment of vision and hearing, irritable colon, isolation (depression), impecunity (money problems), iatrogenesis, insomnia, immune deficiency, and impotence.[14] Many of these problems may become chronic diseases, like diabetes, heart disease, osteoporosis, and dementia. Hopefully, if lifestyle changes are made in early to mid-adulthood, many of these chronic diseases can be avoided or prevented altogether. In our earlier work, we defined successful aging as the avoidance of disease and disability, active engagement with life, maximization of cognitive and

---

12. Thomas Merton, cited in Manning, *Reflections for Ragamuffins*, 259.

13. Geriatric physicians are specialists in the medical care of older adults, like pediatricians are specialists in the care of children. They are particularly well trained to identify medical conditions that can be treated in late life and the multiple problems sometimes caused by chronic illness. They are aware that some medications work differently in older adults than in younger persons and are skilled in identifying potentially harmful drug interaction effects.

14. Kane et al., *Essentials of Clinical Geriatrics*.

physical fitness, and spiritual/emotional growth and maturity. To this we now add "resiliency" because older, successful aging people engage in creative problem-solving as they navigate and treat the chronic conditions that begin to develop in mid- and late life.

Perhaps just as important is a category of assessment for older and disabled people called "functional status." This status helps professionals evaluate a person's capacity for independent living. They may use terms like activities of daily living (ADLs) and instrumental activities of daily living (IADLs). The assessment and problem lists are so long that many may be tempted to deny, ignore, or minimize the risks, but we cannot afford to avoid this discussion. We will talk more about how to meet or avoid many of these specific challenges in the forthcoming chapters, particularly in the chapter on the tasks of eldercare.

Later in the book we will discuss the significance of looking back, using life review. Many have observed that those who do not learn from history are doomed to repeat it. But we live in an era that is increasingly "questioning" history. Sadly, one of my (Mike's) colleagues and a partner with our center, the previous chair of the history department at the University of Alabama, shared that during a PhD oral dissertation defense (examination), five professors in the history department were astonished when the candidate denied the historical accuracy of the Holocaust. "It didn't happen," he claimed. "It is just a Jewish conspiracy to make the Germans look bad." One faculty member took the lead: "You're not going anywhere until you deal with the truth."[15] We need senior faculty in our colleges concerned about the character of our students and more Christian faculty at Christian universities considering using the paideia model of education we discussed earlier, which focuses wholistically on the development of character. Jim and I have never seen such an open, systemic hatred for the Jewish people and the nation of Israel, which is saying a lot for Jim, who was a professor at Oxford during the 1940s, when the Holocaust was largely hidden from the world by the Nazis. Today, the hatred is openly expressed on campuses by university students at Oxford and other public universities like Harvard. As of this writing, the Israeli Defense Forces are defending Israel on multiple fronts with various terrorist groups representing Iran and other nations who do not recognize or observe international law. Christians must courageously stand up and speak truth against cycles of evil, violence, and hate that hinder our ability to learn from history.

15. Clayton, "Port Rail," para. 7.

DISCOVERING THE EXTRAORDINARY AND RECOGNIZING THE ETERNAL

With the apocalyptic event of the coronavirus (COVID-19) pandemic, the severe racial and political unrest, and the invasions of Israel and Ukraine, it is easy to be distracted from ordinary, everyday living. The dramatic aging of our population remains essentially forgotten as one of the world's most important public health issues! But this new book and the James Houston Center are *not* just about what is normal or even what is now being called the "new normal." Rather they are much more about discovering the "extraordinary" in the normal, our "divine potential"! While on sabbatical at the University of Edinburgh a few years ago, I (Mike) discovered a curious note on my faculty sponsor's office door: "The only normal people we meet are people we have just met." There is a certain truth to this statement, but should this be our mindset as Christians when we first meet someone? Perhaps a better approach was taken by C. S. Lewis, who viewed every "normal" person as a highly valued, eternal being. In fact, he went so far as to say that if we could see how the ordinary people of this world will appear in heaven, we would be tempted to worship them![16]

Growing old is a part of normal living for most. One older saint described waking one morning "feeling" old. As soon as she said so, the Lord seemed to say to her, "What did you expect?" We maintain the uplifting truth for some of us that, the older we grow, the more different and wiser we *can* become. We can be better prepared to face whatever the future brings, to include death and what lies beyond the grave. Research shows rather clearly that people become more diverse as they age (e.g., courageous, hopeful, wise, imaginative, kind, disciplined), not more alike, like some of the ageist myths and stereotypes suggest (sick, retired, frightened, lonely, sick, sexless, demented). Jim and I do not want to be tempted to believe that there is only "ordinary" living. But, as C. S. Lewis exclaimed in a wonderful service that Jim was privileged to hear in person one Sunday morning in 1941 at Great St. Mary's Church in Oxford, "There are no ordinary people!" Created in the "image and likeness of God," we are destined to live eternally in an unimaginably glorious future. Lewis's extraordinary comment left Jim

---

16. Lewis, *Weight of Glory*, 15. On June 8, 1941, C. S. Lewis delivered the sermon from which this reference was taken, "The Weight of Glory," which would go on to be one of the most renowned sermons of the twentieth century. Lewis discusses the scriptural meaning of the word *glory* and how it affects us as Christians, both in our earthly lives and into eternity.

standing in awe and wonder of all his human companions, both living and deceased! Therefore, our incentive to be wise is not just for this world, but also for the life to come. One of my (Mike's) older mentors, Dr. Charles Davis, taught me to think about my life as a childlike adventure in Christ: "Michael, we are, in fact, the dearly beloved children of our Abba Father God, and his favor rests on us, and we can trust him"—and, we would add, in this life and the life to come. Our trust then cleaves to this promise that whatever happens in our lives is designed to form Christ in us.

GAIN THE WHOLE WORLD

I (Mike) listened to a remarkable sermon, which I recall as being by Reverend Colin Smith on Moody Radio. Reverend Smith spoke on the profound verses found three times in the Scriptures: "What good will it be for someone to gain the whole world, yet forfeit his soul?" (Matt 16:26; Luke 9:25; Mark 8:36). Now that many have had their "worlds" collapse about them, we think there is some benefit in identifying some of these worlds before we consider the ultimate, all-important question Jesus asks about our souls. Reverend Smith identified the worlds of knowledge, sports, ministry, relationships, leisure, health, vocation, and the arts. All of us have heard messages that address the temptations of our "worlds," and how they can become idols and distract us from what is eternally important.

However, this time Smith emphasized the positive features of each of these eight worlds. With so much wrong in this world, as Christian elders, we can stress the joy of learning and examining the world of ideas, for our heavenly Father most certainly designed us to be lifelong learners. Though I (Mike) am biased and spoiled as a fan of Alabama football, we can all join in the excitement of sports at all ages and levels of athletic events. We can discover the fulfillment of ministry as we work out God's purpose for lives without the artificial restrictions and boundaries associated with retirement.

From a health perspective, we can rededicate ourselves to the welfare of our social convoy of friends and family who are aging in time with us, while we do our best to avoid disease and disability by maximizing our cognitive and physical fitness, knowing that lifestyle often trumps genetics and "wear-and-tear" theories that can leave one feeling helpless. With God's encouragement and empowerment, we can embrace the restorative value of rest and respite, and the inherent beauty and healing that can come from the arts. Just as the Harvard priest Henri Nouwen spent days at the Hermitage in St. Petersburg studying and discovering the depth of Rembrandt's Spirit-inspired painting *The Return of the Prodigal Son*, we can explore our own artistic abilities and affirm those of our children, grandchildren, and great-grandchildren.

As many of us face the collapse of these "worlds" as we know them, Jesus is saying first and foremost that our souls are of infinite value! We also believe that Christians must continue to function as "salt and light" to preserve and restore that which is good in each of these worlds that make up and shape our lives. After all, many of these worlds are part of God's plan to help us learn to "love him and enjoy him forever."

JESUS IS OUR FOUNDATION

The more we learn about purposeful living, successful aging, late-life resiliency, elder caregiving, wisdom, and other topics we cover in this book, the more we recognize how little we can understand, apart from the grace of God, for, truly, everything begins with Jesus. We should not be surprised by this, for he was different than all other men. He was expected: his birth split history in two (the periods before and after his birth), and he came into this world to die. You ask how someone could be wise and come into the world to die? Death was a stumbling block to many like Socrates because it interrupted his teaching. In contrast, death was Christ's aim. His death was not something that happened to him that might have been prevented. Rather, it was the very reason he came. God forgives sin because of Christ's crucifixion. His words of wisdom and love are difficult to understand without keeping in mind his death on the cross. He presented himself as Savior, not Teacher. Bishop Sheen comes alongside C. S. Lewis with a range of alternative characterizations of Jesus: liar-deceiver, insane (delusional, psychotic), or "he was who he said he was," the Christ, the Son of God.[17] Who do you say he is?

OUR INVITATION

If you are a senior, we hope that you appropriate the wisdom of God "that can be ours only through a relationship with the incarnation of wisdom,

---

17. Sheen, *Life of Christ*, 160; Lewis, *Mere Christianity*, 55–56.

Jesus Christ."[18] We hope that you age with wisdom, resilience, and purpose because of your eternal relationship with the King of kings. Whether you are a Christian or not, come, take this journey of aging with Jim and me. Our respective journeys span two lifetimes, though one is a bit longer. Our lives testify to the resilient empowerment of the light of Christ that shines in the darkness. Between the two of us and like many of you, we have been through some really deep waters in different seasons of our lives: a wife of sixty years diagnosed with Alzheimer's disease; a son sustaining a life-changing spinal cord injury; military service in three foreign wars, involving trauma and moral injury; unexpected, parental caregiving duties from a distance; COVID-19, Katrina, and Tuscaloosa's F4 tornado; multiple high-risk career changes to include meeting the challenges of tenure and promotion at a secular, major university; founding a new international Christian college; reacting to a host of concentrated surgeries and iatrogenic experiences; and serving as a Christian scientist at a major secular university studying controversial subjects of faith, spirituality, health, and aging. As we walk together through these and other life- and age-related events and challenges, we hope that you, likewise, will discover the presence of the wisdom that can be known only through a personal relationship with Jesus, the one true source of wisdom in this life and the next. On a personal level, our aim in this book is to add purposeful, resilient "years to your life and life to your years"[19] until that appointed time when you and we are called to our eternal home and our missions in this world are completed.

At the funeral of George H. W. Bush, a contemporary historian described Abraham Lincoln's "better angels of our nature" and Bush's "thousand points of light" as companion verses in America's national hymn. Both Lincoln and Bush were called on to choose the right over the convenient, to hope rather than to fear, and to heed not our worst impulses but our best instincts.[20] To this, Jesus challenges his followers even further in the Sermon on the Mount: "You are the light of the world. A city that is set on a hill cannot be hidden. Nor do they light a lamp and put it under a basket, but on a lampstand, and it gives light to all who are in the house. Let your light so shine before men, that they may see your good works and glorify your Father in heaven" (Matt 5:14–16 NKJV).

---

18. Guthrie, *Wisdom of God*, 11.
19. A common expression in gerontological circles.
20. NBC News, "Meacham Calls Bush."

Chapter 2

Dr. Houston's Stories of God's Providence, Favor, and Purpose

IN DECEMBER 1961, EARLY in my career as an academic, I was on sabbatical from Oxford in Canada. I had just taken ten busloads of InterVarsity students from the various universities in Winnipeg to InterVarsity's wonderful Urbana conference. We came back very moved and challenged in our hearts and our faith by what we heard there, particularly by the missionary appeal. Two nights later as I lay in my bed, I was amazed to see an intense light at the foot of my bed. Oddly, I didn't feel surprised or even curious, simply deeply convinced I was in the presence of God. My response was similar to the reaction that Saul of Tarsus had when he was stopped in his tracks on the road to Damascus and when he saw a bright light: "Lord, what do you want me to do?"

For seven years I waited for the Lord to answer that question. Finally, the answer came. I knew what it was that I had to do: to give up my family's safe and happy life at Oxford and return to Canada. So, in faith, I moved my family. On the ferry crossings from Vancouver Island, I read Søren Kierkegaard for the first time, which opened my mind to new depths of Christian understanding. I still recall sitting on the ferry sundeck, feeling the joy of being a Christian with Kierkegaard as my mentor.[1] God's grace, guidance, and providence would ultimately result in the founding of Regent College in Vancouver.

---

1. See Houston, *Joyful Exiles*.

Regent College is now a well-established graduate school of Christian studies, whose stated mission is to "[cultivate] intelligent, vigorous, and joyful commitment to Jesus Christ, His church, and His world."[2] At any point, about five hundred students are enrolled in full or part-time studies. As of this writing, I would estimate about five thousand students have secured degrees. In any given year, one third to one half of students are Canadian, another one quarter to one third are American, and the remaining 20 to 30 percent come from around the globe. Chinese students make up a considerable proportion of the latter group, whether from the mainland or Taiwan. Hong Kong is home to more Regent alumni/ae than any other city in the world after Vancouver. Regent includes many students each year from Australia, New Zealand, and the UK, with recent students coming from countries as diverse as Kazakhstan, Korea, South Africa, Indonesia, India, Finland, and Brazil. As a result of my act of obedience in leaving Oxford and moving to Vancouver, the Lord has touched the world with the gospel.

Now we turn to Mike's story about the providence of God in his vocational and spiritual life.

---

2. Regent College, "About Us."

Chapter 3

Mike's Stories of God's Providence, Favor, and Purpose

MY FATHER'S DEATH, BORN AGAIN, AND DESERT STORM

At about the ten-year mark in my military career, I had to face my father's progressive frailness. My father was dying. I had an opportunity to spend two weeks with him in the hospital before departing for an overseas military assignment just prior to the beginning of Desert Storm. I remember my departure like yesterday.

My wife, three children, and I were to board a plane within the hour . . . a plane that would take my family and me to another country. Somehow, I managed to recognize the significance of the moment . . . I might not see my father alive again. As my family said their separate farewells, I remained alone with my dad. As I stood next to his bed, I was taken back to a vivid childhood memory. It was bedtime, and I had just slipped into my bed. I must have been about nine or ten years old. As I lay there, my dad quietly entered my room. I know that he must have thought I was asleep, and I was careful to promote that misperception. He leaned over the bed and gently kissed me on my forehead. Like many members of the stoical, World War II generation, my father was rarely demonstrative. I presume that is, in part, why that moment is so meaningful to me after so many years. How I wanted at that instant to return to a childhood time of innocence and safety. Like so many adult children who experience a reversal of roles with their aging parents, I found myself as a father to my own dad. So, I turned to him and said: "Dad, I'm going to do something now that you did for me many years ago when I was a child." I leaned over and kissed him on his forehead. Three weeks later, I learned of his death.

What follows is my memorial to my father, which I wrote on the return flight to his funeral. My father was a well-known businessman who was an elder for over forty years in a large, well-established Presbyterian church. There were over two thousand people at his funeral. My sister was opposed to having my memorial read at the service; furthermore, it would be very unusual for a testimonial like this one to be read at a high Presbyterian church service. Nevertheless, I talked my sister into allowing me to share it with Dr. McClure, my father's pastor. She consented with the understanding that it *not* be read in the service. I was not able to meet with Dr. McClure, so I placed it in an envelope and slipped it under his office door.

Minutes before the service, Dr. McClure placed his hand on my shoulder and said, "Michael, I have decided to break with the traditions of this church, to read what you have written." Before I could say anything, he had entered the church. Needless to say, I hoped it would not be read because my "older" *big* sister was vehemently opposed to sharing it publicly. The first part of the service went well. As I began to ponder my memories of my father, Dr. McClure said, "I am going to break with the traditions of this church and read something Michael has written." My sister's posture reflected her displeasure and alarm, though after the memorial was read, she patted my leg as if to say, "It's OK." Later, she would comment that "it was all in the delivery." Either way, you be the judge. I think my father's memorial underscores two important aspects of late-Christian-life, genuine spirituality: forgiveness and unconditional love.

> I have many wonderful memories of this church. Its influence has been intricately woven into the tapestry of our family. This was the church my father selected for his family. I recall days as an acolyte and as a member of the children's choir . . . vacation Bible school . . . Sunday school. I remember the infant baptism of three of my four children, my own adult baptism, my sister's wedding, and my mother's memorial service. I recall the influence of the Children's Fresh Air Farm (a camp for underprivileged children), and my father's influence on it . . . How he helped the church constructively confront some of the pivotal moral choices concerned with its operation (the acceptance of African American children). And I remember the wonderful support my sister and I received

from this church and its staff in helping my father lovingly make the transition from his home to Kirkwood (an aging-in-place facility). The church has clearly influenced my family for good.

Most of you know that my father's health had become progressively worse following my mother's passing. He suffered without complaint, and he never turned down an invitation to worship here irrespective of his health. His death represents a glorious escape from a body that had become a shell of what it once had been. So we celebrate my father's victory over death. A victory made possible by Christ.

But Christ has done much more for my family. For you see, I was a prodigal son. My father loved me at my worst. How I appreciate that lesson of life as a parent . . . the importance of loving our children at their worst. For I think we all secretly wonder whether anyone could love us in that shadowy condition. Dad's Christlike perseverance with me helped precipitate my own conversion. A few years ago, with all the notoriety surrounding "born again" Christians, I asked my father if he had known any genuine "born again" individuals. In words I will remember forever, he said "You, son!" Those words testify to the miracle of Christ in the life of a family. My father's words symbolized how Christ can reunite families.

"For I am persuaded that neither death, nor life, nor angels, nor principalities, nor powers, nor things present, nor things to come, nor height, nor depth, nor any other creature, shall be able to separate us from the love of God which is in Christ Jesus our Lord" [Rom 8:38–39 KJ21].

> The power of God to change lives
> . . . to give us hope in confronting death.

My father was a multitalented, gifted man with a wonderful dry wit, who lived sacrificially for his family and his church.

We celebrate his entrance into glory today.

God's Providence in My Vocational Calls

I became interested in aging when my father grew seriously ill, and I found myself woefully unprepared to meet the challenges of elder caregiving. I wanted to honor my father in keeping with the fifth commandment, and I wanted to honor my country with military service. Though I made many mistakes as a distant caregiver while assigned overseas, the Lord granted me an unforgettable, memorable farewell with Dad.

After my father's death and funeral, I returned to my challenging overseas position in Heidelberg, Germany. Looking back, I think it was my most complex and demanding assignment. At that time I served as the drug and alcohol consultant to the commanding general of the Seventh Medical Command, which included oversight for six inpatient programs, ninety-five outpatient clinics, thirty-seven adolescent programs, a drug testing lab, and five counselor training programs in Munich. I also served as a member of a European Crisis Action team that was involved in hostage release missions in Lebanon and Syria. I was like some of you who face simultaneously the care of your parents at a high, demanding point in your career. I was deeply touched when my brothers and sisters in uniform found the time to hold a memorial service for my father, for we were in the early stages of Desert Storm and our war with Iraq. At the service, I learned an important fact: I was not alone; many military family members faced aging parent issues, including my commanding general. I would quickly learn that these events were part of God's larger, providential plan and purpose for my life.

After losing my father and learning about others who wanted to honor their parents while serving their country, I felt prompted by the Holy Spirit to pursue postdoctoral, specialized study in aging at the University of Michigan. This redirection would require the grace and providence of God in overcoming some seemingly impossible hurdles. In faith, I applied for a distinguished postdoctoral fellowship as an act of faith and obedience to God's direction and call on my life. I hoped to help other families "get ready" for the eldercare experience that hits most adult children in their forties, often when they are at the apex of their career, like I was. If my vision was true, I felt confident that God could open and close any door necessary, to include my meeting the academic challenges of a postdoctoral fellowship.

The University of Michigan offered a two-year, National Institute on Aging postdoctoral fellowship program, but to attend the world's mecca of age-related, advanced training, I would have to secure permission from the Army Medical Department for long-term civilian training. So, I faced two immediate hurdles, both requiring the grace and favor of God, followed by a third. Once the University of Michigan selected me, my faith increased, and I felt my career direction was affirmed. Then came a serious hiccup. I was told later by my military colleagues in psychiatry, all of whom outranked me, "Parker, we are a young army! So we are recommending to the commanding general that you complete a child and family fellowship at Walter Reed Army Hospital." Acceptance of such an appointment would have been a career-enhancing honor. It was hard to turn down, but I had heard from my heavenly Commander. When I declined this career assignment, I was promptly told that I was placing my career in jeopardy . . . i.e., over! Now God would need to act. Someone suggested I talk with my boss, a two-star general, who, at the time, had responsibility for providing medical care for Desert Storm, a war that was being fought for the first time in American military history by units already deployed across thirteen nations, in what we called the European theater of operations. Saddam Hussein had released death squads into Europe to blow up our hospitals, schools, and living quarters. My children went to school under armed guard for protection, and our quarters were surrounded by armed guards.[1]

Objections Overruled

The general had the weight of the world on him, for we had already deployed the Eighty-Second Airborne and were concerned about their vulnerability until other troops could be sent. Seventh Medical Command was concerned about the projected casualty rate if Saddam Hussein utilized chemical and biological weapons we thought he possessed. Our casualty calculations were of great concern. Nevertheless, sensing that God was with me, I scheduled an appointment.

First, I thanked him for coming to my father's memorial service. During the first few minutes, he mirrored the words of my colleagues in psychiatry. Then he opened the door. He asked what I planned to do at Michigan, and I told him that I wanted to help military families be prepared to address aging parent issues. I reasoned, "If we require soldiers to complete a family care plan prior to deployment (i.e., they may not come back), then do we not also need to help soldiers get ready for caring for their aging parents?" His entire countenance changed. He shared how he had just received a call from his family priest. "I just came from your mother's home," the priest had said, "and she didn't know the gas on the stove was on. What do you want me to do?" The general looked at me and said, "I didn't have a clue what to tell him, but you tell those *** people who are opposing

---

1. Most of the "armed guards" had not been given ammunition, but the enemy did not know it, as far as I know.

your assignment to the University of Michigan that I support you." I never told anyone anything, but the next day my colleagues congratulated me for "sticking to my guns." So, rather than my facing the "end of my career," God opened a door. After the war, I was reassigned to the University of Michigan and my professional life changed dramatically—all in keeping with the Lord's plan, I think, and the fifth commandment.

When the war ended and we returned to the US, my wife took me to Rome, Georgia, to visit my father's prep school, Darlington, where there were records about my father's history. Perhaps they could answer questions I had about my father's life. In a matter of moments, thanks to a diligent director of alumni services, I learned important things that I had never known about my father—things of which I could be proud. This was so important to me in gaining some closure, for we did not always get along because of my prodigal lifestyle as a teen. He had had a scholarship to Georgia Tech, which he did not take because he had needed to work for his family's sake. The onset of refrigerators virtually eliminated what had been a thriving family ice business. He had served on the school's honor council, maintained an A average in his classes, played five musical instruments, and held the national record in the hundred-yard dash (10.4). He also had smoked picayune cigarettes, which eventually got the best of him. Oh, how I wish I could have asked my father more questions about his life.

Please consider using the AgeReady program offered later and online to capture your parents' stories.[2] This information about my father was a part of his story, and it blessed me and my entire family, much like in the Old Testament days, when elders would "intentionally" bless their children. Jim and I heartily recommend John Trent, Gary Smalley, and Kari Trent Stageberg's book, *The Blessing*. Now we promote church-based, life review programs that encourage aging individuals and their families to capture their stories. Someone once said, when an older person dies, it is a bit like burning down a library. Our hearts are broken when we are too late to capture their stories, like with thousands of seniors who died alone in nursing homes of COVID-19 without their families present, or those who no longer remember because of dementia.

After finishing the postdoctoral fellowship program with the help of outstanding mentors in aging,[3] and later, after completing other duties with the military, I felt God's clear prompting to transition once again from a

---

2. See www.beageready.com.
3. Drs. Andrew Achenbaum, Ruth Dunkle, Berit Ingersoll-Dayton, Toni Antonucci.

military to an academic research career in the field of aging. But would an academic position be available? At a bit past midlife in age, I turned down in faith a promotion and another excellent assignment with the then-called Army Health Promotion Command, and I joined the faculties at UAB School of Medicine and the University of Alabama as a tenure-track assistant professor (like becoming a second lieutenant again). Both ran interdisciplinary centers on aging with some of the top researchers and faculty in the field of aging. The director of UAB's Center for Aging and Division of Gerontology, Geriatrics, and Palliative Care was Dr. Richard Allman, a dedicated Christian geriatrician who was forming his center and department of geriatric medicine on the "Michigan model," the very program I had just completed! Accident? I think not.

After a few years at the University of Alabama, by God's grace, the Gerontological Society of America selected me as one of the Hartford Foundation's Geriatric Scholars. The foundation provided additional training and important funding for the development of a "parent care readiness program," which was tested at the US Air War College. Through these marvelous programs and opportunities, I became personally linked to leading scholars in different professions across the world in the field of aging. As things unfolded, I could see God's providential plan at work.

After completing twenty-three years of research and teaching in the field of aging, I felt God's prompting again to launch the James Houston Center for Faith and Successful Aging. The Lord provided one of Birmingham's leading businessmen, who leads us today. Our center has some of the world's top leaders in the field of aging who serve as partners.[4] As I look back on my life, I'm convinced that the Lord has had his hand on me and my family. Who could have known that God would have led someone like me into the field of aging to work with so many marvelous professionals representing an array of professions, like the world-famous theologian Jim Houston, all committed to the welfare of seniors and their caregivers.

---

4. See https://www.jameshoustoncenter.com/partners.

II. Our Spiritual-Emotional Side

Chapter 4

Prayer as Friendship with God

PRAYER, QUITE SIMPLY, IS God's way of enabling communication between himself and us. It is his invitation for us to meet with him, and not only to share our thoughts but also to listen to him.

PRAYER IS FRIENDSHIP

Prayer is living in the presence of a loving God. It is so natural that we do not need the technical mindset of "how to pray" but live in imitation of the One who demonstrated prayer. This relationship with God is a two-way relationship that goes both vertically between us and God, and horizontally between us and others, for prayer evokes community. Having been created in the image and likeness of God, we are intrinsically relational beings. We have been made to desire friendship with each other as well as with God. As such, prayer is the way we shape our inward life to imitate the mind of Christ, and with prayer, with friendship, comes obedience. "You are my friends if you do what I command" (John 15:14 ESV). Ultimately it is a battle of the will. The battle makes us choose whom in the end we really want—God or ourselves.

As we enter prayer, we prioritize our relationship with God. The medieval monks had a rhythm of prayer and work, *ora et labora*. Prayer came first and set the rhythm and priority of God before and in all else. Their work then was an expression of their relationship with God, not some adjunct and onerous task to complete. When we prioritize the relationship, prayer becomes a joy, a necessity, like air is to our lungs. It no longer is seen as a checkbox item done before the day begins or before a meal is eaten, but is an ongoing walk with God, our Redeemer and Friend. It is important that we pray consistently, as the day begins, but, as with any of our human friendships, an ongoing connection is vital. We take time for formal prayer, but we are aware of God's presence with us throughout our days. God invites us to take everything to him, to share whatever is on our hearts. He is a true Friend of friends.

PRAYER AS A WINDOW FOR THE SOUL

As in any relationship we can face the discomfort of true self-knowledge. That is why so many people live with masks, afraid to show others their true selves. They are afraid to face even their own self, to see themselves as they truly are. So, the evasion is to live behind a wall of lies. Prayer is the mirror to the soul and cuts across all pretensions. Lies cannot be expressed in prayer. If we thought our mothers had eyes in the back of their heads, seeing all the naughty things that we did when we were young, how much more clearly does God see and know us! It takes humility, but that humility leads us to pray more for our real needs and teaches us how to approach God. As we know ourselves, we find we cannot afford not to pray and to confess. Augustine, one of the great early fathers of the church, knew this well. He wrote *Confessions*, which exposed his former life, while being a bishop of the church. His church robes were no cover before the Almighty God, and so he penned the beautiful prayer "Lord Jesus, let me know myself and know Thee, and desire nothing save only Thee."[1]

Self-knowledge that we gain through prayer as God shines his light on our hearts demands humility. Anselm, a great medieval scholar, reputedly expressed this dilemma that we all feel with such knowledge of ourselves:

> Oh painful dilemma!
> If I look into myself, I cannot endure myself.
> If I look not into myself, I cannot face myself.
> If I consider myself, my own face appals me.
> If I consider not myself, my damnation deceives me.
> If I see myself, the horror is intolerable.
> If I see not myself, death is unavoidable.

---

1. Augustine, *Confessions*, 187.

Self-awareness and humility lead us to face the realities of sin, as we stand before the righteous and holy God. Yet in that awareness we come to ask: ask for forgiveness, ask for strength, for patience. It also becomes the place to receive: to receive his forgiveness, acceptance, and love.

PRAYER AS A HEART ATTITUDE

Prayer is not something we "do" but a heart attitude. It is not a routine recitation of words and structure that is mindlessly spoken, but true communication of both giving and receiving, from the heart. God seeks to know us intimately and to know the very core of our being, our heart. Prayer is the pathway by which we explore a deeper and more intimate relationship with God. The psalmist David asked of God: "Search me, O God, and know my heart; test me and know my anxious thoughts. See if there is any offensive way in me, and lead me in the way everlasting" (Ps 139:23–24 NIV).

Through prayer we develop as whole people before God. We are as God intended when, in prayer, we are open; we confess; we have been forgiven, cleansed, humbled, sustained, guided, strengthened; and are daily renewed and inspired.

As our starting place is our own hearts, we may find obstacles in praying. These may arise from broken human relationships, wounds from childhood that color our perspective of God, or undealt-with emotions that become directed at God. Yet, trusting in what God says and not in how we feel, acting in obedience to the call to pray, to be in communion with God, will lead to God's Spirit showing us his truth and love. God is offering us friendship out of a gift of love. He transforms us through prayer, and we become new, the unique people who he intended us to be.

PRAYER AND COMMUNITY

As our relationship with God grows through prayer, we cannot help but share that relationship with others. So, prayer builds and is built by community, the horizontal aspect of prayer. Just as we need the friendship with the Trinity, we need the human friendships that encourage spiritual life through all the highs and lows of earthly living. The apostle Paul is a great example to us of his love and appreciation of his spiritual friends who not only benefited from his example, but who also fed and encouraged him. Paul's teachings have great depth and character partly because of his own experience in prayer and suffering. His friends were with him in the dark of a jail cell and sat with him through the difficult times. Dietrich Bonhoeffer remarked in *Life Together: The Classic Exploration of Faith in Community* that none of us can afford solitude if we do not live in community, nor can we have real community without solitude.[2] Solitude with God allows for inward growth, which is enriched within the community of friends. This is the place where we live out the inward work that is being done.

PERSONAL EXPERIENCES OF PRAYER

Prayer, being a relationship, cannot be squeezed into a compact box of understanding. It is often better understood through experiences of others. My father (Jim's) modeled prayer for me when I was a little child. He prayed for all our needs, often on his knees through the night, praying for our morning breakfast. God provided, although it was not always in ways in which we had specifically asked. As a growing Christian I always felt intimidated by my father's example, feeling that prayer was never going to be my forte. However, discovering that it wasn't a technique, and getting to know the personal God, I found that prayer was simply my friendship with my Heavenly Father. I found my own personal rhythm, and, as with my parents, prayer was central to my home life with my wife and children. I had personal and intimate times with God but also family, community times. We celebrated and wept together in prayer, sought guidance and wisdom as a family, and struggled through our hurts in the Spirit. Just as my father taught me and I have taught my children and grandchildren, God is faithful and will never leave us. My desires are not only for navigating the complexities of life but much more so to discover an ever-deepening communion with God. Nine years ago, my wife passed out of this world, and yet, when I am praying, I feel closer to her than I ever have. She is simply through the veil with Jesus, and my closeness to him leads me to closeness to her. Prayer is the conduit.

As a senior now in a full-care home, I (Jim) live in a community of others who otherwise might not cross my path. It is my joy in the long, quiet days to continue to pray not only for my family and friends but for those with whom I now live. I have opportunity to speak words of hope and kindness to a community who daily and more poignantly face death. My bodily struggles give opportunity to use gentleness and kindness to a

---

2. Bonhoeffer, *Life Together*, 17.

physiotherapist who works my tired and sore body. "Breathe in thankfulness, breathe out kindness." My breakfast companions may be seeing the end of life with loneliness and futility, or are lost in a world of dementia, yet their personhood is not lost to God. As I meet with God, he gives me strength to see as he sees, to love as he loves, and to show compassion as he shows compassion. My spiritual companions spur me on to love more deeply and to care more broadly as they love and care for me. We have been equipped to be a channel for God's love and light in the world. Through his power and presence, he uses us to bring his kingdom on earth as it is in heaven.

Prayer is essential! It is in prayer that I grow to know him and thus know myself more deeply; and as I know myself, I know God more deeply. It is in prayer that I see others in his new light, and in communion with others, I am encouraged and uplifted as God works differently in their lives.

Chapter 5

Learning to Dwell in His Presence

Places of Prayer

And when you pray, you shall not be like the hypocrites. For they love to pray standing in the synagogues and on the corners of the streets, that they may be seen by men. Assuredly, I say to you, they have their reward. But you, when you pray, go into your room, and when you have shut your door, pray to your Father who is in the secret place; and your Father who sees in secret will reward you openly.

Our Father in Heaven, hallowed be your name. (Matt 6:5–6, 9 NKJV)

Very early in the morning, while it was still dark, Jesus got up, left the house, and went off to a solitary place where he prayed. (Mark 1:35 NIV)

I (Mike) struggled initially, as a non-theologian, to write this section on prayer without first making sure that I had something substantive to share, given Jim's two scholarly, well-received books on the topic. As I thought about it, prayer has helped me have a sense of his presence, while navigating some of life's greatest challenges, storms, and choices. My marriage to Lane was a clear manifestation of God's grace, for Lane had been engaged to someone else, on my recommendation, no less. The church was a bit surprised when she changed the name of the future groom but not the date, though many in the church had been praying for this outcome.

Virtually all the literature I reviewed highlighted the importance of prayer, though many authors conceded that they found it difficult. I found Dwight L. Moody's sage advice and wisdom helpful in approaching the topic: the two first essential means of grace are the word of God and prayer . . . emphasizing that these two means of grace must be used in the right proportion.[1] If we read the word and do not pray, we may become puffed up with knowledge; and if we pray without reading the word, we may be ignorant of the mind and of the will of God.

BIBLICAL EXAMPLES OF ANSWERED PRAYER

Many do not pray because they think God does not answer prayer. Biblical writers have testified broadly about how and when God has delivered his people. Abraham of the Old Testament was a man of prayer, and the angels came down from the heavens for a chat with him. We know that Elijah brought down fire on Mount Carmel, after the prophets of Baal had failed in their prayers to do so; Elisha prayed, and life came back to a deceased child. The wicked king Manasseh cried out to God from captivity in Babylon, his cry was heard, and he was returned to the throne in Jerusalem. Near the end of his life, Samson prayed, and his strength returned; in desperation, Job prayed, God's favor returned, and his estate was restored. Daniel prayed, and Gabriel came to tell him that he was a man greatly beloved of God and the secrets of God were imparted to him—God's Son was going to be cut off for the sins of his people. Cornelius prayed, and Peter was sent to tell him words by which he could be saved and delivered. Peter prayed, and he saw a vision of a sheet coming down from heaven. Paul and Silas in prison at Philippi prayed and sang, the place was shaken, and the jailer was converted. Stephen at the time of his death looked up and prayed, the heavens opened, and the Son of Man was seen. How wonderful God is to us when he hears our prayers and responds to them.

Of course, the greatest example of the importance of prayer is Jesus our Lord, who prayed to his Father at every major decision point like the selection of his disciples and the feeding of the five thousand. At his baptism, Jesus prayed, and the heavens came down. He prayed at his transfiguration, and his countenance changed, and his clothing turned dazzling white (Luke 9:29). Jesus prayed all night before delivering the Sermon on the Mount and at the grave of Lazarus before raising him from the dead (John 11:41–42). He prayed before his crucifixion, knowing he would make atonement for all our sins (John 12:27–28).

---

1. Moody, *Prevailing Prayer*, x.

PRAYER AND AGING

So, what does prayer have to do with successful aging anyway? Well, our research and that of many others suggests that older people have higher degrees of spirituality than other age groups and that they tend to pray more often than younger believers. Some visionary colleges, realizing the benefits of the old befriending and teaching the young, have placed senior housing and programs on college campuses. When most older people find that they are a part of a young believer's social convoy, sometimes linked to them through social media, they help protect themselves from loneliness and minimize the risks of having only similarly aged people in their social convoy (like attending a lot of funerals).[2] While at the University of Alabama, I thought we could help jump start an anti-ageist movement across the campus by setting a university-wide policy that the old could attend the university gratuitously. These kinds of intergenerational efforts can help older people avoid loneliness and gain a sense of late-life purpose, while the young often gain an older, wiser friend who will pray for them.

A few years ago, I had the honor of serving as the president of the West Alabama Retired Officers Club. Many of our members were veterans of World War II, including some retired officers who served with the famous Tuskegee Airmen. We managed, for one of our banquets, to match up many of our World War II vets with ROTC cadets from the University of Alabama. As a result, many of the cadets established genuine friendships with their older sponsors. Perhaps greater vision is needed to explore other ways to harness this engine of intercessory prayer available from those dwelling in long-term facilities. Even those who suffer severely with one or more of the dementias, depending on the stage of development of the disease, can benefit greatly by remaining involved and connected to the activities of the church as long as possible, like preaching, teaching, sharing with others about their experience, singing in the choir, and being involved in prayer groups in some manner.[3]

Jim has edited one book and written another on the importance of prayer, both of which I heartily recommend, because they emphasize, among other matters, the eternal value of deepening our friendship with

---

2. See the aging-in-place program at the Spires, Berry College, Rome, Georgia (https://www.retireatberry.com/life-at-the-spires/berry-connection/). In return, the young have someone who will pray, befriend, and mentor them.

3. Everman et al., *Dementia-Friendly Worship*.

God through prayer.[4] I will never forget a recent discussion I had with Jim about prayer. I had just shared with him the rather comprehensive organization of my regular morning prayer time, to which he simply shared what he prayed for that morning. "Mike, as I was praying this morning, the Holy Spirit brought to my mind a young, persecuted, Chinese Christian for whom he wanted me to pray." He prayed expectantly, and the Lord directed his prayer time.

A GLIMPSE AT PRAYER IN A MEGACHURCH

A well-known pastor of a large, modern megachurch promotes the biblical idea of praying *first* before practically all activities and decisions. He thinks Christians of all ages should cultivate a lifestyle of prayer in several ways. Each New Year, thousands of his church members commit to twenty-one days of morning prayer (from six a.m. to seven a.m.). Throughout the year, members of his church also gather every Saturday morning to pray for the requests the church received the previous week. Though I had attended Billy Graham meetings, gatherings of men at Promise Keepers conferences, Faith and Successful Aging conferences, and early morning prayer breakfasts, I had never witnessed thousands of people of all ages praying so early in the morning across twenty plus church campuses located in different cities. The pastor of this church thinks that many Christians want to pray more, but don't know how to do it. In response to this need he wrote a prayer guide that covers a range of topics.

On a personal level, the lead pastor encourages his members to have daily prayer, when possible, at a certain time, at a certain place, and in a certain manner, what many modern Christians call their "quiet time," modeled after Christ, who often sought out quiet places for prayer to his Father.[5] Using the Lord's Prayer (Matt 6:9–13), the tabernacle prayer, warfare prayers, and the prayer of Jabez (1 Chr 4:10) in the prayer guide, he gives alternative models of prayer that can be used and tailored to one's spiritual needs. In addressing a broad range of needs, he provides Scriptures that can be prayed that cover confession, forgiveness, pride, generational bonding, healing, marriage, racial reconciliation, intercessory prayer, and other personal issues.

---

4. Teresa of Avila, *Life of Prayer*; Houston, *Transforming Power of Prayer*.
5. Hodges, *Prayer Guide*, 4–5.

When I (Mike) pray in solitude, I make an effort to pray out loud, on my knees, the scriptural promises (Rom 8:15). During the day I ask the Holy Spirit to help me to pray often, pray first, and pray continually to discover his purposes for our lives.[6] Sigmund Freud may have believed "pleasure" was the primary motivation of adults, but Victor Frankl, a survivor of the Holocaust, having never lost a patient to suicide, believed that finding purpose in later life and engaging in purposeful living were the keys to being fulfilled.[7] Fortunately, a growing number of older Christians are seeking to discover where God is moving in the world. For example, Jim and I believe that God is allowing people to live longer for his purposes. So, we need to know his will and to seek to do it. I have tried to pray intentionally about decisions, big and small, and at times of great need, when the Holy Spirit has provided clear, unmistakable guidance in three ways: through fellow believers, alignment with his word, and an opportunistic change in circumstances.

PERSONAL PRACTICES OF PRAYER

At the closing of the Sermon on the Mount, Christ spoke about how a house built on the rock can withstand the storms of life: "Everyone who hears these words of mine and acts on them will be like the wise man who built his house on the rock. The rain and the floods came, and the winds blew and beat on that house, but it did not fall, because it had been founded on the rock" (Matt 7:24–25 NRSVA). During my four careers (twenty years on active duty, twenty-three years of academic life at a major university, a third career with a nonprofit, and twenty-two years as a caregiver to our quadriplegic son), I have gradually incorporated the habits of prayer used by three prayer warriors—Christians I have come to admire: Eric Liddell, the great, Scottish Olympian and missionary; Elisabeth Elliot, the courageous missionary, speaker, and writer; and Amy Carmichael, caregiver and missionary to India's orphans and victims of the sex trade.[8]

I have used Eric's structure for my daily prayers, which served him well for most of his adult life, including his period of captivity by the Japanese during World War II, and when he had much of England angry with

---

6. See Blackaby et al., *Experiencing God*, 35.

7. See Frankl, *Man's Search for Meaning*.

8. The movie *The Sound of Freedom* is helping to expose the epidemic nature of the sex trade problem today (see Monteverde, *Sound of Freedom*).

him for refusing to run in the Olympics on the Sabbath. Elisabeth, wife to martyred missionary Jim Elliot, was a courageous prayer warrior. Ultimately, she and her daughter went to live with and shared the gospel with the tribe that had murdered her husband. I have some of her quotes and favorite Bible verses in my notes that I use every day. I heard her speak, and I have adopted some her approaches to prayer. Finally, Elisabeth Elliot wrote a wonderful biography of the remarkable missionary Amy Carmichael.[9] Amy founded an institution to help Indian orphans and the child victims of the sex trade of her day in India. She cared for so many orphans and received so many requests for prayer that she found she could not keep up. So, she began the practice of praying the name of each child, knowing the Lord knew everything about each child already.

SYSTEM OF PRAYER[10]

Regarding my prayer time, I try to set apart a minimum of thirty minutes in the morning, before others are up and about, in our library, our prayer room. I try to read aloud the Scriptures that I am studying and some of the following verses and reflections.

Christ's guidance:

"And when you pray, you shall not be like the hypocrites, for they love to pray standing in the synagogues and on the corners of the streets, that they may be seen by men. Assuredly, I say to you, they have their reward. But you, when you pray, go into your room, and when you have shut your door, pray to your Father who is in the secret place; and your Father Who sees in secret will reward you openly" (Matt 6:5–6 NKJV).

As part of my daily prayer, I remind myself every morning who God is to me. God is my source, a shield about me, my sun, my deliverer, my fortress, my stronghold, my shepherd, my rock, my higher place, my righteous tower, the lifter of my head, my glory, my strength, my song, my stay, my good shepherd, my salvation, my keeper, my fortress, my stronghold, my all.

When someone asks me for prayer, I try to pray with that person at that moment.

---

9. Elliot, *Chance to Die.*

10. Please forgive me if I sound like a legalist, but I found I needed the structure. Perhaps something I share will truly embellish our own approach.

Throughout the week:

I pray for my family daily;

I pray on Monday for my work;

I pray on Tuesday for extended family members;

I pray on Wednesday for friends;

I pray on Thursday for ministries we support;

I pray for authorities in the nations, particularly those that persecute Christians.

LIFE VERSES

- For the Lord God helps Me, / Therefore, I am not disgraced; / Therefore, I have made My face like flint, / And I know that I will not be ashamed. / He who vindicates Me is near. (Isa 50:7–8a NASB 2020)
- God, be merciful to me a sinner! (Luke 18:13 NKJV)
- This Book of the Law shall not depart from your mouth, but you shall meditate in it day and night, that you may observe to do according to all that is written in it. For then you will make your way prosperous, and then you will have good success. (Josh 1:8 NKJV)
- Search me, O God, and know my heart; / Try me, and know my anxieties; / And see if there is any wicked way in me, / And lead me in the way everlasting. (Ps 139:23–24 NKJV)
- Give ear to my words, O Lord, / Consider my meditation. / Give heed to the voice of my cry, / My King and my God / For to You I will pray. / My voice You shall hear in the morning, O Lord; / In the morning I will direct it to You, / And I will look up. (Ps 5:1–3 NKJV)
- Let the words of my mouth and the meditation of my heart / Be acceptable in Your sight, / O Lord, my strength and my Redeemer. (Ps 19:14 NKJV)
- But You are He who took Me out of the womb; / You made Me trust while on My mother's breasts. / I was cast upon You from birth. / From My mother's womb / You have been My God. (Ps 22:9–10 NKJV)
- [The Lord's mercies] are new every morning; / Great is Your faithfulness. (Lam 3:23)

ERIC LIDDELL'S DAILY PRAYER QUESTIONS[11]

- Have I surrendered this new day to God, and will I seek and obey the guidance of the Holy Spirit throughout its hours?
- What have I specially to thank God for this morning?
- Is there any sin in my life for which I should seek Christ's forgiveness and cleansing?
- Is there any apology or restitution to make?
- For whom does God want me to pray this morning?

PERSONAL ANSWER TO PRAYER

I can remember seeking God's help in granting me favor with my dear future wife, Lane Knudsen, now my wife of forty-six years. The power of prayer and God's grace were interwoven in our love story. At one point during our early friendship, Lane asked me if she should accept the engagement ring from a man I did not know. "I guess so," I said. Sometime after this, I spoke with a girlfriend about Leo Tolstoy's Christian faith, as expressed in his classic *War and Peace*. I was so disappointed in the lack of spirituality in my girlfriend's response that I took a risk and called Lane. We talked late into the night. When I woke up the next morning, I knew in my heart that I was in love with Lane, a stunningly beautiful, brilliant woman who had never made a B in all her years of study and who had graduated first in her senior class of nine hundred. I was a bit intimidated. Now what to do? She had taken my earlier advice and was now engaged to this other fellow. Before my Christian conversion, I would have tried to manipulate the circumstances in my favor.

Little did we know that everyone at church and our places of work was praying that Lane and I would get it right. As I reflect on what happened, I realize that earlier in the year, I had asked Lane to help me start our church's first intergenerational small group with an eighty-year-old retired Presbyterian minister, Reverend David Simpson. As an enthusiastic, newly born-again Christian (May 27, 1976), I sought counsel from my now-eighty-one-year-old friend, Reverend Simpson, and our associate pastor, Tony Dean. We also belonged to an intergenerational Bible study group. Reflecting on those days, I now think Tony helped orchestrate my

---

11. See the questions throughout Caughey, *Eric Liddell*.

relationship with Lane. He had asked us to co-teach a young adult Sunday school earlier in the year. When I told David and Tony of my newfound love, both counseled, "You have to tell her. Then, Mike, you have to pray and wait." After much prayer on both our parts and sound biblical counsel from an older saint, Carrie Rutledge, Lane broke off her engagement with the other man. Some church members were dismayed, wondering why the date of marriage remained the same, but the name of the groom had changed. It is clear that we were surrounded by older Christians who proved to be very positive influences on us and our decision to marry.

As I share some of the stories of my prayerful encounters in my prayer closet with God, and how I have tasted repeatedly of his love and provision, I hope you will sense how God has rescued my family from harm; delivered and redirected our careers; blessed us with four adult children who are strong believers; and given us five grandchildren and three great-grandchildren. My faith has steered me through many challenges, including the Spirit-led decisions to complete a postdoctoral fellowship in aging at the University of Michigan and to change the direction of my career from the military to an academic research career in aging.

Hopefully the stories I have chosen about my own life and that of others, including some uncommon Bible heroes and characters, will inspire you to run, not walk, to our Abba Father for fresh vision, direction, and purpose irrespective of your age. Our primary purpose in this chapter is to inspire you in your own pursuit of a deeper friendship with God through prayer.

PRAYER AND TRAGEDY

For me (Mike) prayer at its best has become a lifeline, like a walkie-talkie[12] to God on the battlefields of life. Perhaps my use of warlike terms (e.g., battlefield) is not the best, but let me share just one from a number of examples of how this thinking has worked its way into my ideas about prayer. For me, the difficult circumstances of my life have often been beyond my control.

I learned a lot about prayer twenty years ago. At two o'clock in the morning we received a call from a UAB-trained neurosurgeon telling us our son was entering surgery for a fractured spine, that he would likely be paralyzed and would be rendered a quadriplegic for life, if he survived a saltwater drowning and the spinal surgery to follow.

12. *Walkie-talkie*—A device not unlike a modern-day cell phone with limits.

My wife and I cried out in desperate prayer that our oldest son, Mike Jr., would survive his drowning and fractured spine (C5–C6). The circumstances were beyond my control, and I felt absolutely helpless to help my son. I'll never forget the kindness of two dear Christian friends (Drs. Roff and Klemmack) who offered their car and necessary cash and spiritual support. Our son survived the surgery. During his inpatient rehab that followed, we formed a parent prayer support group that met regularly. Many of our prayers were answered. After his inpatient rehab, our son moved back into our home, which had been transfigured to accommodate his disability. Our master bedroom was converted into Mike's den, which would later be called the "Bear Bryant Room." I remember one night, shortly after his return home, Mike managed to throw himself out of his bed and began banging his head on the floor. As I embraced him, I prayed for God's presence and help as I would learn to do often during his times of suffering. Since the early days of his injury, Mike has experienced some remarkable answers to prayer. He received a scholarship, graduated with honors from the University of Alabama, started his own TV show on Alabama football, and basically fulfills the role of cool uncle with our grandchildren. Most importantly, he recently accepted Christ as his Savior and was baptized, with friends and family looking on.

PRAYER WARRIORS

I (Mike) was fascinated as a child with study of great soldiers and the battles they fought. Later, after the ultimate battle for my soul ended with my conversion, I became enamored with Christian prayer warriors. One soldierly story is worthy of honorable mention because it serves as an example of the invaluable, incalculable importance of prayer in giving us the courage to follow God's direction at moments of great opportunity. General Joshua Chamberlain, Union hero of Gettysburg, was selected to receive the surrender of General Robert E. Lee and his army at Appomattox, effectively ending the Civil War. The night before, Chamberlain prayerfully decided, at risk of court-martial, to call his thousands of troops to a soldier's salute to the remaining, surrendering Confederate Army. General Gordon, the surrendering Southern commander, also a Christian, was shocked at first. Then he quickly realized the honor Chamberlain was bestowing on his troops. Raising his horse up, he bowed and touched his sword to his boot.

This single act of kindness helped sow the initial seeds of peace after four years of unfathomable, intense conflict.

As a career soldier, I often moved. Now that my children are adults, I am learning more and more about the sacrifices they made as members of a military family. The first thing I did when moving into military quarters or civilian housing was to locate my prayer closet. As Christ advised, I always found a quiet place. Now it is located in a small library next to the front porch of our home, where the morning sun often sheds its light upon me. I like having around me all the great books I've accumulated since becoming a Christian in May 1976. On the wall above the spot where I kneel for prayer is a small, oil-painted version of Rembrandt's *Return of the Prodigal Son*. I also like to fast and pray during retreats to our cabin located in the wilderness of the Appalachian Mountains, where I have sensed the presence of our Abba Father God. I have tried to establish the habit of prayer as a lifestyle the Lord has allowed me to cultivate. I often pray at midday and evenings in the small chapels located on military installations and college campuses. Once I went to sleep in a military chapel, only to be awakened suddenly by the military police, who fortunately recognized me. When praying in the chapels over the years, I search for the pew with the greatest light on it.

THE VALUE OF PRAISE AND WORSHIP

During Desert Storm and during the Vietnam War, I had occasion to be called into a "war room," where generals and senior commanders shared intelligence and made decisions that affected the lives of service members and their families. The war room was a solemn, somber, no-nonsense place. Briefings were made and critiqued, and the information was often contested. After my Christian conversion, I began the practice of an early morning "quiet time" when I read the Scriptures and prayed. Over time my prayer room took on the appearance of a war room, like the ones I had known during Desert Storm . . . a place where questions were asked, plans were made, and decisions were made.

WONDERFUL PRAYERS

The Lord's Prayer:

> Our Father, who art in heaven,
> hallowed be thy name;
> thy kingdom come;
> thy will be done;
> on earth as it is in heaven.
> Give us this day our daily bread.
> And forgive us our trespasses,
> as we forgive those who trespass against us.
> And lead us not into temptation;
> but deliver us from evil.
> For thine is the kingdom,
> the power and the glory,
> for ever and ever.
> Amen.[13]

The full Serenity Prayer, which follows, has been a lifesaver to many who have battled "thorns in the flesh":

> God grant me the serenity
> To accept the things I cannot change;
> Courage to change the things I can;
> And wisdom to know the difference.
> Living one day at a time;
> Enjoying one moment at a time;
> Accepting hardships as the pathway to peace;
> Taking, as He did, this sinful world
> As it is, not as I would have it;
> Trusting that He will make things right
> If I surrender to His Will;
> So that I may be reasonably happy in this life
> And supremely happy with Him
> Forever and ever in the next.
> Amen.[14]

---

13. See https://www.churchofengland.org/prayer-and-worship/worship-texts-and-resources/common-worship/common-material/lords-prayer.

14. Reinhold Niebuhr, "Full Serenity Prayer," in Hazelden Betty Ford Foundation, "Serenity Prayer."

Elisabeth Elliot, the well-known writer, remembered many of the foreign missionaries who stayed with her family when she was a child, but one prayer stood out, the prayer of the Stams.

Betty Scott Stam and her husband were missionaries to occupied China in World War II, and they were both beheaded by a Japanese officer shortly after return to occupied China. Elisabeth remembers praying this prayer with the Stam family before they deployed. This missionary couple was "all in"!

> Lord, I give up my own plans and purposes, all my own desires, hopes and ambitions, and I accept Thy will for my life. I give up myself, my life, my all, utterly to Thee, to be Thine forever. I hand over to Thy keeping all of my friendships; all the people whom I love are to take second place in my heart. Fill me and seal me with Thy Spirit. Work out Thy whole will in my life at any cost, for to me to live is Christ. Amen.[15]

---

15. N. Wolgemuth with Kroesche, "Betty Scott Stam," para. 4.

Chapter 6

Maturing in Holiness

INTRODUCTION

Unlike God, we all have a beginning, and we all have an end. We face mortality, and I (Jim), being over one hundred, face that end more poignantly. The apostle Paul reminds us of the assurance that death has no victory; in the death of Christ, it is swallowed up (1 Cor 15). With that as our finish, how do we live and grow to a "good" end? As Christians we know that life is a daily "dying" to the Lord Jesus: "We face death every day because of Jesus. Our bodies show what his death was like, so his life can also be seen in us" (2 Cor 4:11 CEV). It is a life where daily we give up our own desires and choose to obey the words and examples of Jesus. We may have begun the journey in our early days of Sunday School, or it may be a journey entered into later in life, but we all are on this journey to mature in holiness. Here is my advice for those who wish to mature in this way:

1. Start with the roadblocks.
2. Map out your own unique journey.
3. Live in the Scriptures.
4. Develop the "double knowledge."
5. Practice the presence of God.

1. Start with the Roadblocks

You and I cannot live the faith of our parents; it must be our own unique journey of faith. But ironically, even the faith of our parents can be a roadblock to our growth. That happened to me, for as a "faith missionary" in Spain, my father was often on his knees early in the morning, praying for bread for his children's breakfast. I saw and admired my father as a giant with a strong, persevering prayer life. Yet I was paralyzed in my own prayer life; I could not compete with Dad! So, for years, this was my roadblock. I could not practice prayer in my "quiet time," for I was ashamed I had nothing to report. I dreaded the question "How is your prayer life?" It was empty! I needed to let go of my desire to imitate my father and to have the same kind of prayer life as he did. I needed to allow God to develop my own faith, all the while still learning from and admiring my father. Take time to ask God to reveal the roadblock in your life.

2. Map Out Your Own Unique Journey

In my late teens, I stumbled across the phrase in Luke's Gospel "Lord, teach us to pray." Yes, Lord, teach me! Gradually, it came to me that personal prayer is like one's fingerprint; it is what is uniquely yours and mine. I had always been a lonely child, craving friendships. Then the Lord revealed to me by the Holy Spirit, prayer is simply the cultivation of friendship with God; that's all, yet it is everything imaginable! This aspect of friendship with God became a crucial point in my maturing. While I could learn from others about their relationship with God, each of us has a unique and personal relationship that is tailored for our own personality. We are not to seek to be just like another, but to develop our own relationship with God. Years later that insight led to me to write a book entitled *The Transforming Power of Prayer: Deepening Your Friendship with God*.

In prayer retreats with students who were struggling to know how to pray, I then began to advise them the following:

- Take a sabbatical from prayer—stop trying to pray! For we may have bad habits that need to end.
- Don't start by reading books on the prayer lives of great saints, like Augustine, or Calvin, or Jonathan Edwards! You are likely to remain paralyzed by your admiration of them! You can't imitate them! Allow

- the Lord first to do his work in you and give you a foundation, and then learn from them as examples.
- Allow God to build a new appetite for his presence, and slowly begin to have a daily walk with the Lord.

Gradually, the inner landscape will begin to open new vistas of desire for God's presence with you all the time. It will become your unique fingerprint with God.

3. Live in the Scriptures

As I desired for the Lord to teach me to pray, I spent several months just meditating on the Lord's Prayer. I became so familiar with it that it felt a part of me! For I had begun to realize the Lord's Prayer is not just the words of Jesus, but the human life of Jesus; he embodies the prayer. From there I began to read the Psalms each day, starting at Ps 1, the entry gate of the Psalter, which is all about being "right" or "righteous" before God, and with each other. It is not the language of the way of sinners, cynical and sarcastic. It is truthful and transparent, confessing what I really need and express. The psalmist depicts this entry as like an irrigated garden in a land of drought, needing to receive the water of life to become fruitful. This becomes my springboard to which I constantly return as I read through the Psalms, the songs of the Israelites.

Living in the Scriptures is living in the very words of God. He fills us with his Spirit, and as we listen to his words, we are guided in his direction.

4. Develop the "Double Knowledge"

This is where the great mystics as lovers of God can inspire our journey through life. It was Augustine of Hippo who articulated the desire and prayer: "Let me know Thee, O God, and let me know myself!"[1] This was reechoed throughout the following centuries, so that John Calvin begins his *Institutes*: "The knowledge of God and the knowledge of oneself, in large measure constitute the nature of the Christian religion."[2] A wonderful exemplar is Teresa of Ávila (1515–82), the reformer of the Carmelite

---

1. Augustine, *Confessions*, 17.
2. Calvin, *Institutes*, 44.

Order. The order had been established by women nurses accompanying the soldiers on the First Crusade to the Holy Land, in the thirteenth century. They ended up staying on Mount Carmel to pray, inspired by the prophet Elijah, who prayed against the pagan god of Baal. As Elijah's successors, the Carmelites lived a life of incessant prayer, being also discalced (shoeless), to live the vow of poverty.

Teresa's great classic, *The Interior Castle* (1577), was written at the request of her nuns, to teach them to pray. For Teresa, prayer was simply living in the presence of God by daily dying to oneself. She saw this in seven stages, like mansions of the castle of one's soul, becoming closer to the throne room of Christ as the King of kings and Lord of lords. In summary, these are:

- Prayer for self-realization before God
- Prayer for self-recollection, concerning the character of God and the need of self-surrender
- Recognizing the deception of a good, even exemplary life, that is still self-centered
- Beginning to have a personal encounter with God, as the prayer of silence, quietly aware of his presence
- Prayer of simple, yet intimate union with Christ
- Prayer of betrothal to Christ, which now becomes indescribable since no other love can surpass his love and presence
- Prayer of eternal marriage, with all of one's life, death, and resurrection, now totally transformed to being "in Christ"

Inspired by such saints of God, I (Jim) spent years meditating and lecturing on a series of exemplars of the Christian life.[3] They became life's classics in the communion of saints, just as the ancient classics expressed the heroic life of the ancient Greek identity. These, now I saw, describe the Christian identity.[4]

As we enter this double knowledge of knowing God and knowing ourselves, we become aware of emotional woundedness. Many of us are now aware that in the tenderness of our own childhood, we received relational wounds. Our compensation of them has shaped our personality, positively

---

3. These are collected in the series Classics of Faith and Devotion.
4. See Houston and Zimmerman, *Sources of Christian Self.*

or negatively. When I speak of this to couples, one may deny all this, but the spouse may smile in response, "Yes, dear, it's what I have long called your 'bad breath'!" How many divorces have been caused by the conflicts of one wounding the other by their relational wounds!

I (Jim) have found in my old age, I will get much closer to my children if I explore how I wounded them in their childhood, and that I should pursue adult friendships with my adult children. Even in what may seem very positive ways, we may do this "wounding." We have "high expectations" for a brilliant child, so that they feel a prisoner to parental expectation. We do not give basic trust to a child, wondering later why they became cynical in life, abandoning their trust in God.

A horrendous issue today is the damage from sexual abuse of children. All around us are divided families, where parents ignored the reality within their families, only to face extreme anger and alienation for not knowing or recognizing what was going on to wound a child so deeply. A friend, herself a skilled family psychotherapist, suddenly realized in her forties that she had been abused by an uncle in her childhood. The recovered memory was like the force of hot lava from a volcanic magma plug; the pain was so intense, she phoned me in desperation. Mercifully, she went to an emergency clinic to receive treatment, and is now more effective than ever in her Christian calling.

I (Mike) remember one of the bravest women I've had as a client. She was a Navy wife and mother of young children, who was referred to me by her primary care provider for marital discord. Within the first five minutes she said, "I've had so many affairs I cannot remember them all. And my father molested me in the worse possible ways from age nine to my mid-teens, when I told my mother. He was forced to 'get help,' but he told me privately, 'Unless you let me continue, you can no longer call me your father!' So, the abuse stopped finally, and I left home as soon as possible. And I've never told anyone this about this before." She brought up the issue of the presence of God. "And I ask you, Doctor, where was God when my earthly father was hurting me? Why would I believe in a god who did not help me?" I remember praying, and what follows is some of what I told her in that first session.

I knew that this was a profound opportunity to change how she thought of herself, but if I did not get this right, I knew she would not come back to our military mental health clinic. Looking her squarely in the eyes, I said, "How long are you going to agree with your father about who you are and what you are about? Every time you have sex with anyone but your husband, you are agreeing with your father about who you are and what you are about. The problem is that your father was a liar. The truth is that there is no one else in the world just like you. You are meant to do wonderful things with your life that no one else can do, and you are a blessing to your family and friends!" And the affairs stopped. I transferred her to a group therapy session for women, which was cochaired by a woman. Over time she began to heal and mature, and she and her husband worked on their issues. She developed a strong belief in God, and she began to make a difference in the lives of other women with similar histories.

We face this woundedness through the double knowledge of knowing God and knowing ourselves. "We grow up in every way into Christ our Lord." Various tragedies have deeply taught me, never take the woundedness lightly, but learn and grow through it, for self-knowing before God, in a deeply loved relationship, is life-giving and also lifesaving!

5. Practice the Presence of God

We see great examples of this in the lives of early spiritual leaders. Brother Lawrence, the humble Franciscan monk, inspired the practice as he, the cook in his monastery, tossed the pancakes for morning breakfast.[5] Then in the next generation, the Jesuit spiritual director Jean Pierre de Caussaude wrote letters about this becoming a daily practice to the doubtful in faith.[6]

At the beginning of Christianity, the apostle Peter speaks of the human distinctive as being through "the living and abiding word of God" (1 Pet 1:23 ESV). No other creatures sense or give "presence" as humans do. Yet humans themselves are only a presence to other human beings as they are a presence to themselves. That is, they reflect the reciprocity of full attention, which is love. Their attention, one to the other, is "all there." Only a personal God can be the origin of such divine presence, and only persons in relation can share that.

The early father Irenaeus observed that God cannot be treated as an object, nor can he be known as such.[7] It is his divine presence that draws our full attention as his creatures before the Creator, or as sunlight is before plants in their growth. Uniquely then, we pay full attention to God, for

---

5. See Lawrence, *Practice of the Presence*.
6. See Rohr, "Time-Tested Wisdom."
7. See Briggman, "Irenaeus."

his presence is universal and everlasting. That is why the ancient Israelites carried the tabernacle in their midst in their forty years of wandering in the wilderness; God's presence was in the ark of the tabernacle. St. Benedict stated: "We believe the divine presence is everywhere" (RB 19:1).[8] God's divine attention demands our full attention, because it summarizes the vast mystery of the incarnation, of Emmanuel, "God with us." His divine presence as Father, Son, and Holy Spirit transfigures everything, and it transforms our lives. A new dynamism enters our souls, so that "finding God" is an endless "seeking God."

In my own stages through life, the older and physically weaker I get, becoming more dependent on other people's loving care, I find the consciousness of God's presence grows richer and deeper. As I sleep at night, God's presence in dreams become more important, more inspiring, more directive, for the day's conscious life.

Meeting people has become a daily sense of being attentive to their presence and, reciprocally, being a presence for them. It is now a longtime habit of being in inner prayer, while listening to the needs and sorrows of others. Then one finds that the words shared are effective in comfort or in wisdom. The Eternal "I Am" has become one's universe and one's personal environment.

Our maturing in holiness is a lifelong process. We start with recognizing and dismantling some roadblocks and being aware of the need to recognize our own personal and unique journey. As we live in the Scriptures, hearing more and more the words of God, we come to the double knowledge of knowing God and knowing ourselves. None of this is a flat linear progression, but rather a constant looping and interweaving, as the Holy Spirit leads us to a deeper and more consistent practice of the presence of God. We eventually move to a place of not only a structured prayer life, but also a constant living in the presence of the Eternal "I Am." Maturity is not an instant fix in a fast-paced world, but a slow, gradual, and ever-moving shift toward being whole children of God, his friends.

When I was teaching at Oxford University, I had two students and three faculty colleagues who committed suicide from depression. Their tragedies mark us for life. I also mourn the suicide death of our church organist a few years ago. Her skill as a church musician inspired our worship so deeply. I sensed her depression and tried to reach out to her, but when I was abroad in Brazil, she ended her life!

---

8. Chittister, *Rule of Benedict*, 89.

These tragedies have deeply taught me, never take depression lightly. It can be deadly.

Yes, and self-knowing before God is life-giving and also lifesaving!

> He stilled the storm to a whisper; the waves of the sea were hushed.
> (Ps 107:29 NIV)

The voice of the Spirit is as gentle as a zephyr, so gentle that unless you are living in perfect communion with God, you never hear it. The checks of the Spirit come in the most extraordinarily gentle ways, and if you are not sensitive enough to detect His voice you will quench it, and your personal spiritual life will be impaired. His checks always come as a still small voice, so small that no one but the saint notices them. . . . Whenever the Spirit checks, call a halt and get the thing right, or you will go on grieving Him without knowing it.[9]

And if I go and prepare a place for you, I will come again and will take you to myself, so that where I am, there you may be also. (John 14:3 NRSVUE)

---

9. Chambers, "Quench Not the Spirit," paras. 1–2.

Chapter 7

A Respite in the Storm

A Place for Miracles

I (Mike) cannot think of anyone who, from time to time, has not needed a place of respite. Recognizing this truth is part of successful aging. It helps us navigate the challenges of life while developing resiliency. When I was reassigned to another military installation, one of the first things I'd try to do was to seek out places to go for respite, prayer, and peace, both in my home and at work. At my home, I try to go to my safe room, currently a small library for my daily quiet time, surrounded by my books, a cross-stitched sampler with the greatest commandments (Matt 23:37–40), the antique furniture from my grandmother's county home, an upright piano, an oil copy of Rembrandt's *Return of the Prodigal Son*.

When at work, I can usually find a place of worship, an unoccupied chapel or church where I can "be still" and alone with the Lord, and pray. I realize that some of you may not be able to afford a place for individual and family retreats, but it may be worth making it a line item in your budget. These places of rest have ministered to us. Our cabin on Yellow Creek fulfills such a purpose. We have many amazing stories about what happens when we have gone there with others.

I share the following story that occurred at our cabin because it constitutes, by my standard, a miracle. I think part of aging well is believing that God is still in the business of accomplishing miracles. In some ways, every salvation is the story of the most personal of miracles. As you will see by the following story, miracles can suggest that God is watching and rescuing us in our foolishness. I like to think that God laughed as he rescued me one cold night in my underwear.

At the center of faith is the divine encounter. Certainly, the disciples are an example of the effects of encountering a risen Christ. Shy, uneducated men were transformed by their experiences with Jesus after his resurrection. This transformation is often given as evidence of the reality of Jesus's divine nature. Sixty-five percent of American adults report encounters with the supernatural, and 49 percent have had mystical moments.[1] If you have had such an encounter, why not take the time to capture your encounter for your grandchildren? If interested, read more on the topic in chapter 8, "Life Review," and in chapter 13, "AgeReady," on family domain tasks. Why not share your story with your family and friends?

This is a story of encounters between God, a man, and his dog, and it represents a raw, unexplainable miracle that I witnessed alone, I thought, with one of my golden retrievers.[2] It occurred on a cold, wintry night in December on Yellow Creek in the backwoods of north Alabama. This experience was an epiphany to me in that it helped me to understand better how the Lord chooses to operate. It describes the patience and mercy of God with a man who was close to making a foolish, life-threatening decision. Simply stated, God rescued me, as he has many times, but this was a bit different. And I have not forgotten it. In fact, the story lives on within the hearts and minds of my five (and counting) grandchildren and now, hopefully, you.

During a critical period when our first book was being written, I sought the solitude that our cabin provided. Jim and I were engaged in a battle with our enemy in putting together our book. We had different styles of writing. I had a history of publishing journal articles and refereed chapters of professional books. Having been Oxford trained, Jim writes and thinks a bit like one of his friends, C. S. Lewis. I needed a safe place to listen, think, and write.

At that time, the only way to cross the river to our cabin was by canoe. I had never seen severe weather at the cabin like this before. Snow was falling, waves were cresting, and logs were floating dangerously unrestrained down the river. Armed with a recently written chapter (on the topics of

---

1. Moritz, "Are Spiritual Experiences," para. 1.

2. I think this story is a partial argument for how our heavenly Father uses animals in this world for his good purposes, and if he uses animals in this fallen world, how much more in the heaven to come.

death and dying) from Jim Houston, I prepared myself for the challenge of paddling our two-seater canoe across several hundred yards of the river to our cabin.

The memories of time spent with family and friends help make the cabin a familiar, welcoming place. Not so much this night. It is not some grand structure, but a simple cedar cabin with grand views of nature, the Appalachian Mountains, and Yellow Creek, a tributary of the Black Warrior River. With little to no light, I slid my canoe into the river. As was my custom, I was accompanied by one of my wonderful golden retrievers.

Minnie, the retired matriarch of four generations of goldens for the Parker family, was my trusted companion on this evening. As I think back, I am certain that my heavenly Father was ordering my path, even to the point of orchestrating which dog I took on this adventure. Traditionally, Minnie would swim across the river next to my canoe. Despite the frigid, freezing temperature, as was accustomed, Minnie boldly followed my command to swim the river. Of all our goldens, she had the thickest coat and was most acclimated to the cold. Almost immediately my conscience was quickened with how foolish and insensitive my decision was to this dear animal and friend, who had a long history of kindness to me and many others.[3] Blind to the risk to Minnie and later to me, I let a tradition dictate the moment, irrespective of the sub-twenty-degree (Fahrenheit) weather swirling about us. After she and I made it to the cabin side of the river safely, the words came to mind, "Blessed are the merciful." I felt a bit like Job must have felt when he asked God one too many questions: "Job (Mike), gird up your loins like a man!" Thinking that I had a clear bead on God's theology for the moment, I resolved on my return trip across the river to take Minnie back safely in the canoe. Cold to the bone, Minnie and I entered our cozy cabin as quickly as possible, and I settled down to read Dr. Houston's latest essay for our first book on aging.

Losing a sense of time in my father's reading chair, I realized that I would now have to paddle back in the dark to the marina. The only light visible was a small Alabama Power lamp that I could see dimly on the other side of the river. Embarking this time with Minnie safely in the canoe, I paddled hard against the wind. A strong downriver wake made paddling even more difficult, but Minnie helped stabilize the weight of the canoe.

---

3. Minnie was a friend to everyone, including my daughter's little dog, Rocco, who once fell off our deck into the water. When no one else noticed that Rocco had fallen into the river and that he could not swim, Minnie simply retrieved him . . . and brought him safely to shore.

11. OUR SPIRITUAL-EMOTIONAL SIDE

Halfway across, I thought: "Blessed are the merciful; be kind to this old dog." Safely at the marina, I was careful to be attentive to my dear old companion. After I tied the canoe up "securely," I carried Minnie to our car, which was parked on the bluff overlooking the river. Covering her in a blanket, I returned quickly to the dock to put the canoe up, only to realize that the strong wind and current had pulled it loose from its moorings, and it was now eighty yards off the dock in the middle of river, heading downstream!

Standing on the dock in the darkness on that cold winter night, I foolishly decided, as a prideful swimmer, that I would have to swim in the turbulent, frigid water if I wanted my canoe back. I was not about to lose a perfectly good canoe when it was right there, in sight. Since a recent storm had brought logs into the river, diving and swimming freestyle at night was out of the question. Slow as it was, breaststroke was my only option if I was going to avoid colliding with the logs floating down the river. I considered the risk of hyperthermia, but my stubbornness reigned. As I began stripping down to my underclothes, I counted the cost of such a swim. Embracing our enemy's distorted, false theology, I reasoned that I deserved this cold-water swim. I could just hear the Lord saying, "If you hadn't forced that good, old dog to swim across this cold river, you wouldn't have to experience what old dog did."[4] I felt so alone. But seconds before jumping into the cold, dark water, the word *wait* came gently into my consciousness. I am certain it was the Holy Spirit, partly because it is how the Holy Spirit is described in the Scriptures. I no longer felt alone; instead, I sensed his presence, which was there all the time, anyway.

Within seconds, the canoe that was being pulled downriver by a powerful current made a 180-degree turn directly toward the dock on which I was standing. It was miraculous, given the blustering wind and raging river I faced, that the canoe was heading my way. When it was within thirty yards, I was tempted to swim to it again, falsely reasoning that, though God had saved my life, he still wanted me to taste the same cold water Minnie had experienced. But our heavenly Father was not going to punish me for my foolishness and unkindness to my dog. In a bit of panic, I thought, "What if the canoe turns back downriver?" I would have missed my opportunity! But when God saves, he saves indeed. I didn't have to swim eighty yards, not even thirty, because the word *wait* came to mind again. Somehow, I knew for certain that this time it was the gentle, grace-filled voice of

---

4. In human years, Minnie was in her eighties.

the Holy Spirit. Though I had sensed his presence many times before, this experience seemed unique. Within minutes the canoe butted against the wharf, and canoe, dog, and owner were safe.

Not only had the Lord's intervention saved my life, but I had learned the importance of listening and waiting on the gentle, kind, unobtrusive voice of the Holy Spirit. Second, I learned that he seeks us out in our storms. I checked the landscape for witnesses. Perhaps someone else had seen all of this. Standing securely on the bluff where my car was parked, overlooking the raging river, I literally yelled out in childlike gratitude: "Thank you, Lord, for saving my life!" It was if I sensed a great crowd of witnesses in the heavenlies, so I yelled out like a child, "Hello up there, everybody! Mom! Dad! Mimi, Reverend Simpson!"[5] As I drove home that night, I had a tremendous sense that "others" had witnessed what happened. In Heb 12:1–2 we are told: "Therefore, since we are surrounded by such a great cloud of witnesses, let us throw off everything that hinders and the sin that so easily entangles. And let us run with perseverance the race marked out for us, fixing our eyes on Jesus, the pioneer and perfecter of faith. For the joy set before him he endured the cross, scorning its shame, and sat down at the right hand of the throne of God" (NIV).

Perhaps you have seen the glorious scenes from two of my favorite movies that are all about "finishing well" our respective races.[6] In the final scenes of the movie *Secretariat*, the mighty horse wins the final race of the Triple Crown. In the background, "Oh Happy Day" is being sung by the Edwin Hawkins Singers, and as they sing "when Jesus comes," it is accompanied by views of the joyful faces watching a moment in history when an old horse finished some twenty plus links ahead of his next competitor.[7] Or, you may have watched the movie *Chariots of Fire*. Representing his beloved Scotland, Eric Liddell was a top candidate to win the world's most esteemed race, the one-hundred-yard dash in the 1922 Olympics, but he created an uproar in all Great Britain when he refused on religious grounds to run in the qualifying race on the Sabbath. Imagine if an athlete took such a position today. He was allowed later to qualify for a much longer race. The final scenes of the movie capture Eric winning the four hundred meters with the

---

5. Actually, I know more than four who will be in heaven.

6. One of my dear friends and partners in our ministry to seniors is Hal Habecker, director of Finishing Well Ministries in Dallas. Please visit his website: https://www.finishingwellministries.org/.

7. Wallace, *Secretariat*.

international crowd of family, friends, and fans rooting him home, as Eric says to himself, "When I run, I sense God's pleasure."[8]

Most of us have many races to run. Having recently retired as a professor after twenty-three years of service at the University of Alabama and UAB School of Medicine and earlier as an army officer in the Army Medical Services Corp after twenty years, I am now engaged in another race: to advance the cause of aging Christians and those who love and care for them. Imagine for a moment Jim and I are cheering you home. If you are crossing a stormy river characterized by a lethal disease or a diagnosis of Alzheimer's disease or you are overwhelmed by what you sense God is asking you to do, know that you are not alone. At my retirement dinner at UA, I was asked to speak and reflect on my career. Even though UA is a public university that would prohibit me from talking about my faith, I managed to work the gospel into my lectures by playing both the finishes from the two movies I just described to an audience consisting of largely secular colleagues and friends.

Perhaps some of you appreciated this story vicariously. Or, imaginatively, it reminds you of your own divine encounter/s, which the Scriptures encourage us to share with one another and particularly with the coming generation. If you've had a divine encounter, please consider sharing your story. Reflecting on my own history has reminded me of many other stories that testify of his grace, mercy, love, and providence. These encounters remind me to wait on the Lord in a quiet place and to listen for the voice of the gentle Holy Spirit. Ultimately, in facing death, we wait on the fulfillment of God's promises of eternal life in faith. We can trust God to bring us to shore safely. "Now may the God of hope fill you with all joy and peace in believing, that you may abound in hope by the power of the Holy Spirit" (Rom 15:13 NKJV).

It is hard for me to imagine a smileless Christ in this story. Nor do I see a stern, Pharisaic Christian. I see a joyful Christ with the capacity to erupt in laughter or rejoicing . . . like the parables that often ended with a party

---

8. Hudson, *Chariots of Fire*. Having completed a sabbatical at the University of Edinburgh, Dr. Parker had the good fortune of gaining two wonderful friends, Bob Rendall, CEO of the Eric Liddell Centre, and Maureen O'Neill, director of Faith in Older People, a nonprofit that provides multiple ministries to seniors and their caregivers. Both have become partners for our center. Read more about them at https://www.jameshoustoncenter.com/partners, click their pics, and their bios will appear. Both have a great appreciation of story. Maureen was decorated by the queen of England, and Bob knows the story of Eric Liddell . . . three of my heroes, Bob, Maureen, and Eric. Bob and Maureen have submitted descriptions of their age-friendly programs in the appendices of this book.

or celebration, stories he told of the lost sheep and the prodigal returning home... of being lost but now found (Luke 15:5)! Clearly, celebrations and feasts are in the future of all Christians, if I believe my dear friend, author Kay Bascom![9]

---

9. Bascom, *Jubilee Journey*.

Chapter 8

Life Review

Leaving an Intergenerational Legacy

Examine yourselves as to whether you are in the faith. Test yourselves. Do you not know yourselves, that Jesus Christ is in you?—unless indeed you are disqualified. (2 Cor 13:5 NKJV)

But God forbid that I should boast except in the cross of our Lord Jesus Christ, by whom the world has been crucified to me, and I to the world. (Gal 6:14 NKJV)

But none of these things move me; nor do I count my life dear to myself, so that I may finish my race with joy, and the ministry which I received from the Lord Jesus, to testify to the gospel of the grace of God. (Acts 20:24 NKJV)

Therefore we do not lose heart. Even though our outward man is perishing, yet the inward man is being renewed day by day. For our light affliction, which is but for a moment, is working for us a far more exceeding and eternal weight of glory, while we do not look at the things which are seen, but at the things which are not seen. For the things which are seen are temporary, but the things which are not seen are eternal. (2 Cor 4:16–18 NKJV)

Let nothing be done through selfish ambition or conceit, but in lowliness of mind let each esteem others better than himself. (Phil 2:3 NKJV)

And we know that all things work together for good to those who love God, to those who are the called according to His purpose. (Rom 8:28 NKJV)

Recent surveys of older Christians indicate that many have not discovered God's purpose(s) for their lives. How can this be, given the apostle Paul's encouraging promise in Rom 8:28? How sad this may seem to older people who have less time remaining in this world to make amends for the sins of their past or to contribute afresh to the work of God in this world. Is it too late to make a difference for good? Notable Christian authors and leaders have written books about the purpose-driven life. Pastors of some of the fastest growing churches have emphasized core mission statements about discovering God's purpose and making a difference in this world.

THE NEED FOR REMEMBRANCE

Perhaps one of greatest gifts our elders can give to future generations is to simply take time to examine their lives and tell their unique stories of faith, failure, endurance, and success. Our stories can testify to how God can work all things together for good for those who love God, who are called according to his purpose, just as God did for David (Pss 51, 139), Paul (Acts 9:1–6), Joseph (Gen 50), Esther (Esth 4:14–16), and so many other heroes of the faith (Heb 11). Their stories of God's providence are proclaimed boldly in the Scriptures as stories worth remembering.

Perhaps our final purpose should include capturing our own stories of God's goodness over a lifespan. Sadly, many of our elders have not been challenged to share their unique stories of God's providence in their lives. Jim and I believe that each of us was created uniquely, on purpose and for a purpose, and that we have an opportunity to discover God's call on our lives. We hope that this chapter will help you experience a growing awareness of how important it is that we tell our stories and those of others before they are forgotten.

BIBLICAL REASONS FOR LIFE REVIEW

For the Christian, the purposes of life review and reminiscence help fulfill many biblical admonitions when we capture and share our God-honoring adventures and those of fellow travelers in the faith. In its account of great biblical stories of faith, Heb 11 encourages us to remember our own stories of faith and those of our elders. Jesus often used parables to teach. The lost coin, the prodigal son, the parable of the talents (Matt 25:14–30; Luke 19:11–27) are all stories in the Scriptures that lead us to Christ. Life review provides a Christian with a rich set of methods for capturing his/her own stories and those of his/her elders, which can serve as intergenerational testimonies of God's providence and grace in their lives. In this chapter, we briefly discuss and define life review and reminiscence, contrasting some of the secular theories and biblical admonitions for capturing stories. We also summarize some of the research and ways congregations can institute life review that capture Christ-honoring stories that "boast" of the power of God across the generations.

THE CULTURE

The current cultural Zeitgeist, with its newest technologies, provides people with tempting ways to boast of their "achievements" and secure rather quickly large numbers of social media followers. In Acts 12:21–23, we read the sad commentary on King Herod's life: "On an appointed day Herod put on his royal robes, took his seat upon the throne, and delivered an oration to them. And the people were shouting, 'The voice of a god, and not of a man!' Immediately an angel of the Lord struck him down, because he did not give God the glory, and he was eaten by worms and breathed his last" (ESV). In contrast, a Christ-centered life review and reminiscence can now use modern forms of communication to capture stories that otherwise would be forgotten. These accounts can result in biblically sound, Christ-centered "boasting" of what the Lord has done in individuals. Boasting/focusing on God's work in our lives leads to an honest accounting, spiritual maturity, humility, right living, and a spiritually fruitful life grounded in the gospel. Life review, at the deepest level, can illuminate an individual's source of endurance during times of testing and suffering—the powerful experience of the salvation of the ungodly by faith alone (Rom 4:5), leading necessarily to a life of glorious freedom from a performance-driven life.

USING LIFE REVIEW TO ASSESS PRIORITIES

Life review can help us to counter the deleterious effects of a rushed lifestyle, late-life isolation, dysfunctional family histories, trauma, and racism, all of which are part of a culture of ageism that intensifies the devaluation of older persons. By examining our own lives and by listening to the life stories of others, we can slow down the pace of modern life. Proper storytelling can provide an opportunity to listen to our elders. Their stories can help remind us that God is our refuge and strength, a very present help in trouble. In examining our lives in the light of God's truth, we can lay our load down repeatedly and be reminded to build our lives on God's power and love.

SECULAR BENEFITS OF LIFE REVIEW

From a secular perspective, geriatricians, gerontologists, life course and personality theorists, researchers, oral historians, and clinicians have suggested that varied forms of life review and reminiscence can:

- Enhance late-life awareness of personal accomplishments and unresolved issues
- Preserve the past and give a sense of personal legacy to the future
- Conserve life stories about everyday experiences and special events
- Enhance intergenerational connections across a person's social convoy of relations
- Help a family discover many positive qualities about an older relative
- Prevent or lessen the effects of late-life depression and isolation
- Answer important late-life questions
- Capture the vital world of one person's story with clarity

We recognize that along with life review and reminiscence, other related names and approaches might include storytelling, guided autobiography, legacy work, oral history, life history, life story, creative writing and other forms of artistic expression, memoirs, structured reminiscence, positive core memories, and "experiencing life challenges" interview. Life review groups allow church and group leaders to work with specific sets of people, like those facing the end of life, isolated older persons in long-term care facilities, adult children who are serving as caregivers to their parents, aging veterans, and athletes. So, there are many approaches and methods from which to choose that help the church capture the stories of its elders as we are challenged by the Scriptures to examine and review our lives.

MIKE'S FAMILY STORY

We encourage adult children, older Christians, and congregations to start a life review group. Adult sons and daughters (and grandchildren) can record the individual stories of their mothers, fathers, and grandparents. After my father's death, I (Mike) discovered from the archives of his prep school remarkable things about him that I had never known. As I noted earlier, he held the national record in the hundred-yard dash, had a scholarship to Georgia Tech, was on the school's honor council, played five musical instruments, and smoked Picayune cigarettes. Now I regularly wear the emblem of his school on my coat pocket. When people ask about that school crest, I remind them to capture their parents' stories while their parents have the capacity to tell their stories.

SMALL GROUP LIFE REVIEW

In this chapter, we highlight the value of small groups in developing life review ministries. After prayer, we recommend that you organize a small group in your own church or community where you can examine and share your life or capture the stories of others. Groups can be so powerful. Two of the megachurches with which I (Mike) have worked have a foundational principle: "We are a church of small groups, *not* a church with small groups." Large congregations can help partner with smaller congregations by providing resources that support, sustain, and enhance the quality and vibrancy of small groups.

AN EDINBURGH LIFE REVIEW GROUP AIMED AT SHARING THE GOSPEL

Life review groups can help us to present the gospel in powerful ways. In Edinburgh, Scotland, two elders were challenged by their pastor to offer a new service in the middle of the week for older, "unsaved" people. They confided in me their reluctance to do so. They felt it was futile to start a new service in the middle of the week, when the targeted group refused to attend church on Sunday. I suggested the idea of starting a life review group by inviting other older, unchurched, and churched friends to a meeting in which the group members shared their respective life journeys. Younger members of the group from the University of Edinburgh could help capture these stories using modern forms of communication. Another large Sunday school group in Ann Arbor, Michigan, allowed Dr. Parker to "Skype" the idea of life review during their study of *A Vision for the Aging Church*. The class was packed with faculty from the University of Michigan who were committed to "finishing well" and who saw life review as an opportunity to do just that.

LIFE REVIEW GROUP IN AN ASSISTED LIVING FACILITY

In one outreach effort, we organized a life review small group consisting of young, middle-aged, and young-old adult members representing a small congregation and a local megachurch close to a major university. This interdenominational team interviewed old-old (seventy-five to eighty-five) and oldest old (eighty-five plus) residents of a local assisted living facility. Two young adult members of the team were cinematographers affiliated with the University of Alabama. The team utilized the latest technology to video and edit the stories of senior saints with the full cooperation of the insightful leaders of the assisted living facility. After the Christ-honoring elder stories were captured and edited, the completed videos were given to the participants and their families. Later, the intergenerational team processed and assessed the lasting value of the process to them and to those interviewed and their families. The cinematographers' skill in recording and editing the video footage proved valuable, but they also taught other members of the group how to use new cell phone technologies to conduct life reviews. Most of the participants on the life review team grew committed to the idea of developing and sustaining an ongoing life review ministry, as did the leaders of the assisted living facility, who viewed this ministry as a distinctive, positive addition to their program.

LIFE REVIEW AND CREATIVE STORYTELLING

All of us have been greatly influenced spiritually and emotionally by members of the company of Christians with whom we have been associated, and who make up that social convoy of friends and family who are aging in time with us. Surely, like a ship at sea finds safety in the convoy, so we can attest to the value of those who have helped us in our own journey. In the television series *Band of Brothers*, the story of Easy Company's journey from the Normandy invasion to the surrender of Germany is best captured in the words of their commander, who responded to a question from his grandson: "Grandfather, were you a hero during the war?" "No, grandson," he replied, "but I was in a company of heroes!"[1]

We have known many wonderful 1 Cor 13 people whose lives are a living testimony of God's love and grace. In many respects, they have written their stories and legacies into the lives of other people. I (Mike) know of one friend's father who cared for his elderly wife who suffered from Alzheimer's disease till the day she died, without any help from others. We do not recommend such a strategy, because caregiving should not be a solo journey, but because of his isolation, this elderly man had little time to get to know any of his neighbors. His isolation was a result of his caregiving. Still, the neighbors recognized what he was sacrificially doing. When she died, he received notes of sympathy from everyone in his housing complex. His courageous love story was captured and is remembered by his family and his neighbors.

As Jim has shared about his own caregiving journey with his wife, who also suffered from Alzheimer's disease: "This was the most important season of my marriage. I told Rita that I would be her memory. And if I failed at times, I could reassure her that God would remember her." These and other remembrances are a vital part of Dr. Houston's written memoirs, and only one of many reasons why his counsel has been widely sought on this topic.[2]

WRITING A MEMOIR

As noted earlier, writing a memoir is one method of life review. It can be accomplished individually or in a supportive group atmosphere. *On Kitten Creek: Searching for the Sacred; A Memoir,* by Nancy Swihart, is a remarkable, modern-day adventure story of how one family, grounded in Christian love and guided and empowered by the Holy Spirit, developed a Christ-honoring, relational evangelical community of which I (Mike) and my family were the beneficiaries. There are two powerful verses that Nancy fulfilled in her book and life. In Ps 71:18, we are encouraged to "declare God's power to the next generation, His mighty acts to all who are to come" (NIV). In Ps 90:12, we are to "number our days aright, that we may gain a

---

1. Hanks and Spielberg, *Band of Brothers,* 58:30.
2. Houston, *Joyful Exiles.*

heart of wisdom" (NIV). As we read her story, we remembered and reminisced spiritually about our own families and lives and how God's providence was protectively manifested time and time again in our respective journeys and required military moves/assignments. I consider my meeting, mentorship, and deep friendship and collaboration with Jim Houston part of God's great providence in my own life and, therefore, a part of my story.

As I read Nancy's memoir, I thought about my family's first military assignment, which was a journey of faith, and how we were the recipients of the blessings of the Swiharts' (and Bascums') family-run Wellspring ministry to Kansas State University students from all over the world. My family was the recipient of the love of the Swihart and Bascum families—a love that endures today. In addition to Nancy's accounts of the spiritual impact the Wellspring ministry had on countless humans, Nancy's heartfelt stories of their family's farm animals can be linked to a real-life Narnia tale and remind my family to be thankful for our own experiences we have had with five generations of golden retrievers! So, for some of us, animals should be included in our stories.

Nancy Swihart has written a life-changing narrative, which is what a good memoir should accomplish. As a retired soldier and professor at the University of Alabama, I was impressed by the Wellspring team's openness to the suggestions of college students, their willingness to simply be present, to listen, and to provide a relational community where young people could see faith in action and participate in real-life ministries. In our research and ministry with aging congregations around the world, we recommend Nancy's inspirational book as an encouragement to older persons of faith to share their own Christ-honoring stories in the form of a memoir and to remind adult children to capture the stories of their parents and grandparents.

Nancy provides insightful suggestions about how to tailor our own personal stories. Her memoir guides us to our Savior and encourages us to fully dedicate our lives to him and the gospel, as it reminds us that God provides, corrects, leads, and answers our prayers and needs. Her book reminds us of the importance of remembrance and teaches us how to pray, and think, the Scriptures. During chaotic moments when their farm animals were not cooperating with their live Christmas story for hundreds of visitors, she found herself praying: "He is in me. He who is in me is greater than he who is in the world. He did not give me a spirit of fear, but of love, power, and self-control."³ After reading her life-changing book, my family was inspired to make broader use of our own cabin for ministry beyond our family and to place more importance on ministry with our children, grandchildren, and great-grandchildren. C. S. Lewis reminds us: "There are no ordinary people, when they are recognized to carry an eternal weight of glory. You have never talked to a mere mortal. Nations, cultures, arts, civilizations—these are mortal, and their life is ours as the life of a gnat. But it is immortals with whom we joke, work, marry, snub and exploit—immortal horrors or everlasting splendors."⁴

CREATIVE STORYTELLING, DEMENTIA, AND MILITARY SERVICE

Creative storytelling can be an artistic method of life review and some moderation of healing from traumatic events, like military experience. Winston Groom, the author of *Forrest Gump*, was my wife's first cousin and a member of my extended family. Most of his readers are not aware of Winston's military service in Vietnam, but everyone who saw the movie or read the book can see how he used his combat experience to create and enrich a remarkable tale that affected millions of people.⁵ One of the actors, Gary Sinise, who played Lieutenant Dan in the movie, is now a tireless advocate for active-duty defenders, veterans, and first responders. In life review research, I and a team of researchers used quotes from *Forrest Gump* to enrich the real-life interviews with three Vietnam War veterans who had never written about their experiences.

In a nonfiction book, *The Allies*, about Churchill, Roosevelt, and Stalin, Groom alludes to his courageous, maternal grandfather (affectionately known as Far Knudsen), who served during World War II in the Merchant Marines, along with his son, Olaf Knudsen (Mike's father-in-law).⁶ Coming out of retirement from his service with the United Fruit Company, Capt. Knudsen (Far) led convoys of US ships bearing critical, life-sustaining supplies to our desperate allies when German submarines and planes were destroying American ships daily. These ships sailed from New York and other American ports to many locations—voyages that were nerve wracking,

3. Swihart, *On Kitten Creek*, 818.
4. Lewis, *Weight of Glory*, 45–46.
5. Groom, *Forrest Gump* (book); Zemeckis, *Forrest Gump* (film).
6. Groom, *Allies*, page number unavailable.

both going and coming. During one voyage, twenty-three of thirty-four Merchant Marine ships were sunk, and their entire crews perished in the icy waters. Olaf accompanied his father on several trips. Part of Olaf's story includes a perilous night when his ship had engine trouble and was left behind, isolated and vulnerable to Nazi submarine attacks. The letters of faith and courage he wrote to his family during that long, fearsome voyage remain a valued part of his family's treasure chest of memories about him and his Norwegian father.

Other examples of creative stories that reflect the personal histories of authors abound. It was not until recently that the effects of how World War I shaped the writings, lives, and faith of J. R. R. Tolkien and C. S. Lewis have been clearly illuminated.[7] We aim to use these tales in helping to unravel the moral injuries that have occurred to many modern-day veterans. The horrors of World Wars I and II, the Korean War, the Vietnam War, and our more recent struggle in Afghanistan, Syria, and Iraq have had their unique cohort effects, particularly evident in the high suicide rates of veterans of the more recent eighteen-year war conflicts. Lewis's Narnia tales of the lion, the witch, and the wardrobe and Tolkien's stories of Frodo, Samwise, and Gandalf provided a creative outlet for the combat traumas that both Lewis and Tolkien experienced in WWI and resulted in the publication of some of the most widely read books in history.[8] Our Houston Center's military team sees life review and the creative arts of music, writing, and painting as a healing avenue for many of our veterans suffering from moral injury, PTSD, and other outcomes associated with the trauma of war. As the characters in these varied stories and tales become personalized, we can begin to recognize God's sustaining power and love through our own spiritual warfare and weaknesses, right to the end of our earthly journeys.

Ultimately, a Christian's story or memoir should be honest and Christ honoring, not self-glorifying. Even if we are able to achieve something significant in our lives, if we are honest, we will come to see that all things truly good are manifestations of God's grace, not our own efforts. In reflecting and reminiscing, we must learn to listen carefully to the guidance of the Holy Spirit in our lives. Pride is but one step away from having its ugly effect on our stories. The Holy Spirit will help us to be kind to ourselves without sacrificing honesty.

---

7. Loconte, *Hobbit, Wardrobe, Great War*.
8. Lewis, *Chronicles of Narnia*; Tolkien, *Lord of the Rings*.

Together, Jim and I have over one hundred years of counseling experience, and we have clearly seen the power of small groups in churches of all sizes. We want to encourage a small group ministry focused on memoir and life review, where, hopefully, members of different generations can help each other share their own story. No one's life should ever be viewed as ordinary or mundane. Traumatic memories can result in what military psychiatrists, psychologists, and social workers now call "moral injury." How we treat trauma, whether self-inflicted or cast upon us by natural and man-made disasters, is critically important. Some life events, like the death of a child, cannot be explained. Like the miracle of the shipyard: the steel parts of a ship do not float; however, when the parts are finally assembled (sometimes on earth, surely in heaven), they are unsinkable.

I have a son who suffered a traumatizing spinal cord injury. I could not begin to approach writing my own story or memoir without including some of the lessons I have learned along our caregiving journey with our son, Mike, who was injured on July 4, 2004, while diving into the Gulf of Mexico. So, to us, and particularly to Mike, Independence Day is a day that carries significance far beyond the national celebrations that typify that holiday. As aging caregivers, our ability to care for Mike has underscored the necessity that my wife and I maintain our own health. My wife, Lane, is (forgive the language) a bad***. At seventy-five and counting, she does pull-ups. Most of all, my son's injury has taught me that our house still stands because it was "founded on the Rock" (Matt 7:27).

Post-injury, Mike came to know Christ, and he continues to discover his life's purposes in sports broadcasting, prison ministry, and being a "rock star uncle" to his nephew and four nieces. When a local judge was dying, his wife was naturally very concerned about his absence of faith. After multiple pastors visited, all without reaching the dying judge with the gospel, his wife called Mike. He rolled his wheelchair into this dying man's bedroom, his Bible in his lap. After the visit, his wife called Mike to say that her husband had just said, "Sweetheart, I know now that I will see you in heaven! There was something real and genuine about the young man." Stories, when grounded in genuine conviction of the storyteller, can produce deep conviction in others because they touch the heart.

Closing

Several years ago, it was revealed that the Rev. Billy Graham met privately with Winston Churchill during a break in his famous crusades in London. Churchill asked that the discussion be kept confidential. After Churchill's death, the Rev. Graham felt free to share the story of his meeting with Churchill. At one point during the conversation, Churchill said, "I am a man without hope." This, of course, prompted Dr. Graham to share the greatest story ever told to a man hungry for the good news of the gospel.[9] So may we help others look back over their lives to share their unique narratives of God's love. For many older people, their stories of God's providence represent the most important gift they can give, but someone must be willing to listen and to capture their stories. Their messages represent intergenerational transfers of wisdom, hope, counsel, and direction.

In Mark 5 we read about the remarkable healing of a man in chains, a chronically ill woman restored to health after twelve years of suffering, and a twelve-year-old girl brought back to life. These encounters with Christ attest to how Jesus loved the outcasts and the marginalized. In these stories, Jesus represents the compassionate God who allowed himself to be interrupted. That sick woman, anemic, weak, probably suffering, like many older people today, from the effects of iatrogenesis (bad medical care), was poverty stricken, ceremonially unclean, and alone, seemingly lost in a crowd, yet still she reaches out in humble faith and touches Jesus's robe . . . just the hem of his garment, "and immediately the flow of blood dried up" (Mark 5:29 ESV). She was healed. And Jesus calls out to her . . . not in shame. Instead, he calls her "daughter"! He not only restores her health but gives her hope and status.

Will you consider starting a life review ministry in your church or community? Many of our senior saints have powerful stories to tell, but our churches need leaders to discover God's call to capture the untold stories of God's seniors.

And so it is that we are called to continue the work of Jesus, to represent a compassionate Jesus, a dispenser of grace to those who are without hope. Yet many of our elderly live isolated lives. Some live in prisons. Some are virtually alone in long-term care facilities. Just as Jesus breaks with the normal protocols of the day represented by the heartless Pharisees, we must reach out to the forgotten, the hopeless, and the discouraged. We believe

---

9. Graham, "Finest Hour 116."

that when we capture their stories, we give our seniors needed status in an ageist world. So, boldly, we encourage you to consider capturing the stories of your parents, grandparents, and great-grandparents . . . our aging prisoners, veterans, and residents of long-term care facilities, before it is too late. In so doing, you will break free of the crowd and our culture that often fails to honor its seniors. Such a ministry will help you move your church from "casual" to "intimate." For our elders' stories can help us to know God, discover sources of our own freedom, and find purpose by making a difference. For those seniors who do not know Christ, perhaps someone reading this chapter will sense God's call to develop a small group life review ministry for grandparents, great-grandparents, aging veterans, older prisoners, nursing home residents, and other groups. By the end of life, most Christians have endured years of suffering, and their stories of courage and perseverance deserve to be told. Christians can be the greatest storytellers because they know the greatest Storyteller of all, Jesus Christ!

> Blessed assurance, Jesus is mine!
> Oh, what a foretaste of glory divine!
> Heir of salvation, purchase of God,
> born of his Spirit, washed in his blood.
>
> This is my story, this is my song,
> praising my Savior all the day long.
> This is my story, this is my song,
> praising my Savior all the day long.
>
> Perfect communion, perfect delight,
> visions of rapture now burst on my sight;
> Angels descending bring from above
> echoes of mercy, whispers of love.
>
> Perfect submission, all is at rest.
> I in my Savior am happy and bless'd,
> watching and waiting, looking above,
> filled with his goodness, lost in his love.[10]

---

10. Crosby, "Blessed Assurance."

SAMPLE QUESTIONS TO ASK THOSE PARTICIPATING IN LIFE REVIEW

Spiritual History

- What is your spiritual story?
- What is your faith tradition?
- Describe how you arrived at your faith or lack thereof.
- Regarding your profession or professions, did you feel "called" to that/those profession(s)?
- If your answer to the previous question was that you experienced a "call," how has the nature of that call changed for you over the years, as you have practiced your profession?
- In what ways have your spirituality and/or your religious beliefs/practices influenced your daily work? Your family? Your health?
- Was your faith helpful during troubled times? Please share how it was helpful.
- Please describe how your private religious practices have helped you cope with tough times.
- How has your involvement with organized religion, like a church congregation, been helpful? Please share stories . . .
- Have you lived a crucified life? Have you done humble things joyfully? For Christ's sake?
- Does the thought of "hardness" draw you to a project or repel you?
- Apart from the Bible, can you name three or four books that have been of vital help to you?
- What refreshes you most when tired?
- Have you ever had opportunity to prove our Lord's promises (i.e., to supply temporal as well as spiritual needs)?
- Can you mention any experience you have passed through in your Christian life that brought you into a new discovery of your union with the crucified, risen, and enthroned Lord?
- How has your congregational membership been difficult?
- How has your faith helped you to mature?

- How has your faith helped you with personal illness or disability?
- How has your faith changed your life for good?
- How has your faith affected your marriage? For good?

Family and Friends

- What is your greatest hope for your children? Grandchildren?
- What is the most important message you want to give your children? Grandchildren?
- Do you have one important message to share with your family or one person in your family?
- What would you want to say to your best friend?
- What is your full name? Why did your parents select this name for you? Did you have a nickname?
- When and where were you born?
- How did your family come to live there?
- Were there other family members in the area? Who?

Personal History—Childhood

- What was the house (apartment, farm, etc.) like? How many rooms? Bathrooms? Did it have electricity? Indoor plumbing? Telephones?
- Were there any special items in the house that you remember?
- What is your earliest childhood memory?
- Describe the personalities of your family members.
- What kind of games did you play growing up?
- What was your favorite toy, and why?
- What was your favorite thing to do for fun (e.g., movies, beach, etc.)?
- Did you have family chores? What were they? Which was your least favorite?
- Did you receive an allowance? How much? Did you save your money or spend it?

- What was school like for you as a child? What were your best and worst subjects? Where did you attend grade school? High school? College?
- In which school activities and sports did you participate?
- Do you remember any fads from your youth? Popular hairstyles? Clothes?
- Who were your childhood heroes?
- What were your favorite songs and music?
- Did you have any pets? If so, what kind, and what were their names?
- What was your religion growing up? Which church, if any, did you attend?
- Were you ever mentioned in a newspaper?
- Who were your friends when you were growing up?
- Which world events had the most impact on you while you were growing up? Did any of them personally affect your family?
- Describe a typical family dinner. Did you all eat together as a family? Who did the cooking? What were your favorite foods?
- How were holidays (birthdays, Christmas, etc.) celebrated in your family? Did your family have special traditions?
- How is the world today different than what it was like when you were a child?
- Who was the oldest relative you remember as a child? What do you remember about them?

Family History—General

- What do you know about your family surname?
- Is there a naming tradition in your family, such as always giving the firstborn son the name of his paternal grandfather?
- Which stories have come down to you about your parents? Grandparents? More distant ancestors?
- Are there any stories about famous or infamous relatives in your family?

11. OUR SPIRITUAL-EMOTIONAL SIDE

- Have any recipes been passed down to you from family members?
- Are there any physical characteristics that run in your family?
- Are there any special heirlooms, photos, Bibles, or other memorabilia that have been passed down in your family?
- What was the full name of your spouse? Siblings? Parents?
- When and how did you meet your spouse? What did you do on dates?
- What was it like when you proposed (or were proposed to)? Where and when did it happen? How did you feel?
- Where and when did you get married?
- Which memory stands out the most from your wedding day?
- How would you describe your spouse? What do (did) you admire most about them?
- What do you believe is the key to a successful marriage?
- How did you find out you were going to be a parent for the first time?
- How did you choose your children's names?
- What was your proudest moment as a parent?
- What did your family enjoy doing together?
- What was your profession, and how did you choose it?
- If you could have had any other profession, what would it have been? Why wasn't it your first choice?
- Of all the things you learned from your parents, which do you feel was the most valuable?
- Of which accomplishments were you the proudest?
- What is the one thing you most want people to remember about you?

Record the key aspects of the answers to these questions using audio, video, or text.

III. Our Aging Minds

Chapter 9

Sleep

I lie down and sleep; I wake again because the Lord sustains me. (Ps 3:5 CSB)

JIM AND I HAVE included some content about sleep to emphasize its importance in the health of our aging bodies and particularly to the health of our aging brains. Although almost everyone would agree that we must learn to sleep well, experts with the National Sleep Foundation indicate that only 50 percent of us over the age of sixty-four sleep the recommended average of eight hours a night. Jim and I have focused on this topic because failing to get enough sleep affects us socially, physically, emotionally, vocationally, and spiritually.

Jim has rarely had difficulty sleeping. I, on the other hand, have struggled with sleep intensely for the past two years. Limited sleep puts us in the crosshairs of several chronic conditions like obesity, diabetes, heart disease, dementia, and a shorter life.[1] We have learned that waste material in the brain, like proteins involved in Alzheimer's disease, is removed from our brains during sleep. Sleep also contributes to heart health, improves our mood, makes us more productive, sharpens our perception, and helps us maintain a healthy weight. The benefits of sleep are increasingly being recognized. Sleep is basic for sustaining a healthy life. If you are like me and have trouble with achieving restful sleep, don't surrender to the notion that sleep problems are a permanent part of your life.

Approximately one in three older people will experience sleep problems or may have a specific sleep disorder. Despite its importance to overall

---

1. Harvard Health Publishing and Marshall, *Alzheimer's Disease*.

health and particularly the brain, the frequency of its occurrence among older people who may be at risk for dementia is often a neglected topic during routine health exams. Some cannot get to sleep, others have frequent awakenings, while others experience early morning awakenings or a combination of all three. Other conditions leading to poor sleep include leg movements, abdominal discomfort, and withdrawal from medication. Some problems with sleep can be associated with aging, like decreased time in deeper stages of sleep. Many individuals face nightly challenges related to their life circumstances. During my military career, I often had seasons in which much was demanded of me, and this naturally affected my sleep. In late life, I am now faced with demanding caregiving duties. For you, it may be your work demands and/or unpredictable caregiving duties that you must address. Before we discuss some solutions, I will highlight some of the differences in late-life sleep habits that are part of Jim's and my own experiences. These differences help to contrast different sleep experiences.

I (Jim) am remarkably well at my age of one hundred plus, and I attribute that to having lots of sleep. I have two hours of sleep every afternoon and ten hours at night. Around 350 BC, Aristotle wondered in an essay just what humans were doing in sleep, and why. Now we have a much clearer understanding. The molecular clock inside our brain cells is adapted day and night to living on a spinning planet, to keep in sync with the sun.[2] Awake, we are recording, and in sleep we are editing. This explains why I often go to bed puzzled about how I should research further, only to awake the next day clarified as to what I should write next. The same is true of prayer. I go to sleep worried about how I should help someone, and the next morning it is clear which procedure I should take.

We can say that as food is necessary for the body, so is sleep the food for the brain. That is why in some cultures, as in Spain, where my (Jim's) parents were missionaries, the afternoon siesta was part of the rhythm of life, suited to the afternoon summer heat, while the cool evening was the time for the main meal of the day. In terms of digestion, this is not good, so a light supper is better for older people. The heaviest meal of the day should be breakfast, to allow digestion to occur slowly through the waking day.

As our culture has developed a faster pace of living, we are sleeping less than in the past. This can be very serious, as anyone who regularly sleeps less than six hours has a higher risk of depression, dementia, anxiety,

---

2. Ruder, "Circadian Rhythms and Brain," para. 7.

stroke, and obesity.³ Sleeplessness can undermine your overall health. One of Jim's favorite texts of the Bible is "God neither slumbers nor sleeps" (Ps 121:4), for during the night God is watching over our needs. Often, when I am worried or troubled about something unresolved, I pray God will resolve it for me, while I am asleep. I (Jim) have found that when I am no longer under stress, I no longer experience nightmarish dreams. Indeed, I begin to have humorous dreams and lighthearted dreams about relationships. While having my afternoon siesta today, I even dreamed of the cartoons I could devise for this book. Awakening, I sensed the publisher might think our folksy approach was going too far! I find that humor can help me sleep.

But you may ask, why do we get creative ideas in sleep? I think it is when we are most passive that we are most receptive to God entering into our subconsciousness. When I am wide awake, my ego is much more aggressive, and I am less likely to hear "the still small voice" (1 Kgs 19:12) of his gentle presence. The Lord knows the fundamental importance of rest and told us as much in the beginning verses of the Bible when he rested after creating the world and the universe. Sufficient, high-quality sleep is integral to our health and sense of well-being and vitally important for older people and their caregivers alike.

OUR BIOLOGICAL CLOCK

As we age, it's common to experience changes in the quality and duration of our sleep. Many of these changes occur due to changes in the body's internal clock. Each of us has a master clock in the brain called the hypothalamus. Twenty-four-hour daily cycles, called circadian rhythms, influence other daily patterns, like when people get hungry or sleepy or alert. As people get older, their sleep patterns change. Sleep problems can disrupt circadian rhythms, which directly influence when people feel tired and alert. Light is one of the most powerful cues for maintaining circadian rhythms.

Unfortunately, research shows that many older people have limited exposure to daylight.⁴ Daylight exposure may be even more restricted for older people who live in nursing homes as well as those with Alzheimer's disease. Changes in production of hormones, such as melatonin and cortisol, may also play a role in disrupted sleep in older adults. As people age,

---

3. See Colten and Altevogt, "Extent and Health Consequences."
4. Harvard Health Publishing and Marshall, *Alzheimer's Disease*, 19.

the body secretes less melatonin, which is normally produced in response to darkness. Melatonin helps promote sleep by coordinating circadian rhythms, which is one of the reasons people take over-the-counter melatonin for sleep problems.

NEW INNOVATIONS FOR IMPROVING SLEEP

Sleep masks can help block out unwanted light while providing soothing background noise that can help a person to sleep. Light therapy glasses give off a wavelength of light that can help regulate the body's sleep-wake cycle. AYO light therapy glasses can help keep a person's circadian rhythms more in sync for a night of restorative sleep. Smart home systems' IFTTT (if this, then that) allow older persons to control heating, lighting, security cooling, and other systems in their home.[5]

SLEEP AND CLEANUP

Sleep increases the clearing of waste from the brain, and both growth and wound healing seem to accelerate during sleep. Impairment in the brain's waste removal system may explain part of the increased dementia risk associated with obstructive sleep apnea. Memory function is closely related to sleep quality. Studies have shown that working memory decreased by over one third when the individual was sleep deprived. Memory seems to be affected differently depending on which part of sleep is diminished, especially deep sleep and dream sleep. Adopting good sleep habits and sleep schedules, optimizing the sleep environment (using recorded sounds of rainfall, waves, waterfalls, storms), and effectively treating any sleep disorders can not only increase energy levels but can decrease the risk of major health crises and increase potential life expectancy.

So, for most of us, the tools are there. Ignoring the necessity of sleep, a fundamental component of our health, is foolish, especially when the answers are within easy reach. I found it helpful to avoid sleep medications (hypnotics or sedating antidepressants), choosing instead some helpful behavioral techniques for improving sleep quality: going to bed at the same time every night, exercising earlier in the day, and avoiding blue lights from the computer and TV for at least an hour before bed. A warm bath

---

5. Orman, *Sleep Well Again*, 20.

followed by some "sleepy time" hot tea while reading a magazine or book usually helped me to find rest. For sleep, I (Mike) recommend a book by the famous J. R. R. Tolkien, *The Adventures of Tom Bombadil*. It is the most boring book I've ever read, guaranteed to turn off your brain and make you ready for sleep. In fact, a colleague, friend, and sleep expert, who served as a neurological consultant on this chapter, recommends it to many of his patients.

LIFESTYLE AND SLEEP

Poor sleep quality in seniors can also be related to the lifestyle changes that often come with aging. For example, retirement leads to fewer hours working outside of the home and possibly more napping and a less structured sleep schedule. Other significant life changes, such as loss of independence and social isolation, can increase stress and anxiety, which can also contribute to sleep issues.

It is generally considered a myth that older adults require less sleep than younger individuals. Many older adults have a hard time getting the sleep they need, but that doesn't mean they need less sleep. The amount of sleep that a person needs can decrease from infancy to adulthood, but this trend appears to stop around age sixty. Most experts advise that people over sixty-five should get seven to eight hours of sleep each night.

SLEEP TIPS FOR SENIORS

Older people can take steps to improve their sleep. These steps often involve focusing on improving sleep hygiene and developing habits that encourage quality sleep. Here are a few tips for getting a better night's rest in your golden years:

- Exercise: Older people who exercise regularly fall asleep faster, sleep longer, and report better quality of sleep. Exercise is one of the best things older people can do for their health. The National Institute on Aging offers helpful tips for exercising as an old person. Be sure to include balance related exercises like tai chi.
- Reduce bedroom distractions: Televisions, cell phones, and bright lights can make it more challenging to fall asleep. Keep the television in another room, and try not to fall asleep with it turned on. Move

electronics out of the bedroom and reserve the bedroom for only sleeping and sex.

- Avoid substances that discourage sleep: Substances like alcohol, tobacco, caffeine, and even large meals late in the day can make sleep more challenging. Try quitting smoking, reducing caffeine intake, and eating dinner at least four hours before bedtime.
- Keep a regular sleep schedule: Remember that aging makes it more difficult to recover from lost sleep. Avoid sudden changes in sleep schedules. This means going to bed and waking up at the same time every day and being careful about napping too long.
- Develop a bedtime routine: Find activities that help you relax before bed. Many older people enjoy having a bath, reading, or finding some quiet time before getting into bed.

Chapter 10

Facing the Epidemic of Dementia
A Present-Day Leprosy?

THE ZEITGEIST—THE SPIRIT OF THE TIMES

During the brief time Jesus walked among his people, we have no known biblical accounts of him encountering a person suffering from dementia. People today are living longer, with chronic diseases, so they are at greater risk for dementia than during Jesus's time. However, the ancient disease leprosy would have been a readily observable condition that Jesus frequently faced. Perhaps we can gain some insights from how Jesus handled such a condition as leprosy. As always, the Son of God brought clarity and light to a fearful situation. In one incident he had little difficulty healing the condition, while uncovering the real sin of ungratefulness.

> Now on his way to Jerusalem, Jesus traveled along the border between Samaria and Galilee. As He was going into a village, ten men who had leprosy met Him. They stood at a distance and called out in a loud voice, "Jesus, Master, have pity on us!" When He saw them, He said, "Go, show yourselves to the priests." And as they went, they were cleansed. One of them, when he saw he was healed, came back, praising God in a loud voice. He threw himself at Jesus' feet and thanked Him—and he was a Samaritan. Jesus asked, "Were not all ten cleansed? Where are the other nine? Has no one returned to give praise to God except this foreigner?" Then He said to him, "Rise and go; your faith has made you well." (Luke 17:12–19 NIV)

We have no doubt Christ could heal dementia and other associated maladies today.

We think there are important lessons to be learned in comparing the religious communities' and society's reactions to leprosy and dementia. People feared leprosy in Jesus's day, and people fear dementia today. Leprosy was misunderstood, and in like manner, dementia is largely misunderstood, which is one of the main reasons for this chapter on dementia. Today, people with dementia, as people with leprosy during Jesus's time, are often separated from mainstream society. In fact, the latest research suggests that isolation and loneliness are associated with higher risk for dementia in the young and the old. Chronic loneliness affects young and old and has been cited by the twenty-first US Surgeon General, Vice Admiral Vivek H. Murthy, as a major health crisis. Research shows that loneliness and social isolation can reduce life expectancy and contribute to adverse health outcomes like depression and dementia.[1] Even the church seems confused about how to address the growing incidence of dementia. Because leprosy was a visible symbol of decay and corruption of the body, the religious leaders of that time must have found it almost natural to treat the disease as a symbol of sinfulness. It was generally thought that sin corrupts a person spiritually, the way leprosy corrupts someone physically. We are not implying that most modern Christians think that dementia is the result of sinfulness, but there is clear evidence of bias and a lack of Christlike compassion for the person with dementia and his/her caregivers.

In this chapter, Jim and I take the stand that a person with dementia has not lost his personhood, regardless of his cognitive status. How do we bring the love of Christ to bear more powerfully on such a widely misunderstood condition?

In Jesus's time, lepers were handled as forgotten outcasts, set apart from mainstream society. At times they were reviled, and they were typically avoided. Those who maintained some contact with their families were often a burden as the disease progressed. While walking the roads of his day, Jesus showed a special affection for the lowly, poor, and humble in heart. As time passed, they became known as ragamuffins, or little poor ones.[2] They were the special objects of Jesus's compassion, and it is that same compassion we hope to share in discovering a cure and supporting people with dementia and their caregivers.

1. See Powell, "How Social Isolation."
2. Manning, *Reflections for Ragamuffins*, 11.

Today, leprosy can be treated successfully with antibiotics. During Jesus's time, there was no cure other than an encounter with Christ, which resulted in full recovery for 100 percent of those suffering. Although there are some lifestyle changes and promising new drugs to treat and slow the progression of Alzheimer's disease at an early stage,[3] it remains a devastating disease without a complete remedy. Just as with leprosy, some dementia sufferers today try to keep it a secret for as long as possible, even though much progress has been made by churches that have developed age-friendly programs for people with dementia and their caregivers.[4]

Many fear that if they are diagnosed with one of the dementias, they will face a nightmarish, slow, progressive loss of their cognitive and psychological capacities, rendering them virtually dependent upon strangers in an expensive long-term facility. For it truly is "the long goodbye" disease. As one close friend, who recently lost his dear wife to frontal lobe dementia, was asked how he was after her funeral, he simply said: "I have been saying goodbye to her for ten years!" Unlike leprosy, which in Jesus's day was largely visible, dementia is now thought to be caused by a sticky material called amyloid plaque, which is clumped up between brain cells, and the twisted threads inside cells are known as neurofibrillary tangles. These are thought in most medical circles to be the hallmark, pathological signs of dementia.[5] Most of the discoveries with dementia have been discovered in autopsies, though that is changing. We want and need cures now for this disease that affects the entire family.

Our purpose in this chapter is to bring some hope and clarity to individuals, families, and churches who want to demonstrate the love of Christ to those living with dementia and to their families. What do you really know about dementia? Have members of your family been diagnosed with a specific dementia, like the most common form, the dreaded Alzheimer's disease? If yes, where should this person live as the disease progresses? In a nursing home? A memory care unit? Or at home? Who provides the long-term care? If the sufferer needs long-term care, who pays for this tremendous expense that has bankrupted many? Who in the family is willing to serve as the primary caregiver?

---

3. The FDA has granted accelerated approval for Leqembi, a new Alzheimer's disease treatment that slows cognitive decline in people with early-stage disease (Harvard Health Publishing and Marshall, *Alzheimer's Disease*, 37).

4. Everman et al., *Dementia-Friendly Worship*.

5. Harvard Health Publishing and Marshall, *Alzheimer's Disease*.

In many respects Alzheimer's disease and other dementias have generated a societal fear reaction to the illness. Dementia is not like cancer. Typically, it results in the total loss of all memory and an eventual incapacity to live at home, with expensive long-term care often provided by a nursing home, away from family . . . the long goodbye. A burden on family, long-term care needed, steadily progressive, feared—yes, people with dementia need our help, as do the families that care for them.

A local gifted physician with multiple medical licenses[6] and I organized a health fair targeting older people and caregivers at a large downtown church. Filled with hope and good intentions, and armed with informative brochures, we expected a significant turnout, especially from the Christian community. However, our confidence proved to be misplaced. Despite the success of a previous church-sponsored Faith and Successful Aging conference, which brought together over five hundred seniors from various congregations, our health fair was poorly attended.[7] The topics, including dementia, failed to generate much interest. Some attendees deemed the subject depressing. One man's dismissive comment at the fair revealed the consequences of such attitudes, as he was unprepared for an Alzheimer's disease diagnosis years later. Ageist attitudes are often subtle and camouflaged. In our first book, we talked about a conversation we had with a local progressive pastor from a liberal church and denomination, where we encountered an unexpected example of ageism. When asked about his church's ministry to seniors, he proudly categorized older people as "no gos, slow gos, or fast gos." When pressed by what he meant by a "no go," he said it was someone unable to contribute. "Like a person suffering from Alzheimer's disease?" I asked. I offered the perspective that a person with dementia presents all of us—family, clergy, and fellow church members—with the opportunity to learn how to love a person who cannot love us back. As Christians, empowered by the Holy Spirit, we can be a source of light, truth, and preservation of goodness even amid the difficulties of caring for someone with dementia.

Jim, known for his theological insights, shared his experiences as a caregiver for his wife, Rita, during her extended dementia journey. He realized that he could serve as her memory bearer, offering comfort and love through the preservation of their shared memories. Jim's example reminds

---

6. Geriatric psychiatrist and neuropathologist Richard Powers, UAB School of Medicine.

7. Parker et al., "Multidisciplinary Model."

us of God as our refuge and strength, assuring us that we are eternally remembered as we face dementia ourselves or have a family member who has directly experienced the disease. Perhaps you, like Jim, live with someone with dementia. Alternatively, you might be a son or daughter grappling with caregiving responsibilities from a distant location, like my own experience while serving overseas in the military. Regardless of the circumstances, we can confront the challenging subject of dementia as a community together.

DEMENTIA DEFINED

In this section, Jim and I aim to provide you with a concise overview of dementia, offer strategies to enhance cognitive capacities for as long as possible, and describe common church services and supports available to individuals with dementia and their caregivers. Dementia is a devastating condition that affects various aspects of a person's mental, social, and physical functioning, progressively worsening until death. People suffering from dementia also face, as do the family caregiver(s), financial and emotional strains. As of this writing, the estimated yearly cost for health care, long-term care, and hospice care is about $355 billion with over $76 billion falling to individuals.[8]

As Christians, we must anchor ourselves in the unwavering promises of God. In the United States, dementia, including Alzheimer's disease, has become the third leading cause of death, projected to surpass heart disease and cancer in the future. Unfortunately, there is currently no cure for dementia.

The term *dementia* comes from the Latin words *de mens*, meaning "out of mind." It refers to a group of symptoms characterized by cognitive deficits that interfere with daily activities and social relationships. The onset of symptoms is gradual and insidious, with the progression of cognitive decline reflecting the impairment of brain cells. The course of dementia can vary greatly depending on underlying disease processes and individual factors.

Given the wide-ranging impact of dementia, assessments, treatments, and interventions must address the whole person, considering emotional, physical, psychological, social, and spiritual aspects of functioning, as well as the strengths, character, and faith of caregivers. With the progressive nature of the disease, advance planning becomes crucial for individuals and

---

8. Harvard Health Publishing and Marshall, *Alzheimer's Disease*, 49.

their family caregivers. Medical and social interventions should focus on developing plans to address current and upcoming challenges.

Dementia in the elderly can be categorized into four main types based on causes and incidence rates: primary degenerative dementia (such as Alzheimer's and Pick's disease), multi-infarct dementias (stroke related), partially reversible dementias (vascular diseases, infections, metabolic disorders), and other neurological disorders (Huntington's and Parkinson's diseases). Alzheimer's disease is the most common cause, followed by vascular-related diseases. Dementia can also arise from various other diseases and conditions, including HIV/AIDS, alcoholism, traumatic brain injury, Creutzfeldt-Jakob disease, Down syndrome, and general medical conditions.

The prevalence of dementia increases significantly with age. For instance, at age sixty-five, only a small percentage of individuals have dementia, but by age eighty-five, the percentage rises dramatically. The likelihood of dementia may reach as high as 50 percent among those over the age of eighty-five, those in the fastest growing segment of the population, the oldest old. Due to the aging of the population, the prevalence of dementia is expected to rise significantly in the coming decades, necessitating increased support for individuals with dementia and their caregivers.[9]

Dementia profoundly affects a person's functional abilities. While memory impairment is the primary characteristic, other cognitive disturbances such as aphasia (impaired speech), apraxia (inability to perform motor functions), agnosia (failure to recognize objects), and executive function disturbances (issues with abstract thinking, planning, initiating, sequencing, monitoring, and stopping complex behavior) are also present. As dementia progresses, memory, judgment, language, and the ability to engage in daily activities deteriorate, often accompanied by behavioral disturbances.

Psychiatric symptoms can accompany dementia, leading to personality changes, depression, anxiety, delusional thinking, and hallucinations. Dementia affects other aspects of a person's life, including emotions, memory, judgment, language, behavior, and daily activities. It is important for older individuals and families, especially adult children with elderly parents, to recognize and respond to these symptoms. Appendix G provides information on Daphne Johnston's faith-based dementia respite program

---

9. Harvard Health Publishing and Marshall, *Alzheimer's Disease*, 3.

for family caregivers, while AgeReady offers a program designed to prepare all caregivers for the challenges of caregiving.

One person with Alzheimer's disease described his experience as the "gradual loss of short-term memory, failure to recognize lifelong acquaintances, terrifying hallucinations, sudden bouts of rage, loss of judgment and awareness of time and place, numbness in the lower limbs, and cancer left untreated as an exit strategy."[10] In contrast is the older person who simply suffers from a slower processing time for new information. Most age-related memory loss does not stem from Alzheimer's disease, but is related to attention and retrieval of information. Memory problems can be related as well to stress or fatigue. Older people may require more time and effort to learn new information, but once they've learned the material, they retain it as well as younger people. In most cases, the earlier a serious cognitive problem is identified and treated, the better.

GOOD NEWS

We have some more good news. The presence of mild cognitive impairment (mild memory impairment) does not always progress to full-blown Alzheimer's disease, and there is some information that would encourage all of us to make some changes in our lifestyles that we can control. While risk factors like age, gender, and family history we cannot control, we can work to control our cholesterol levels, blood sugar, blood pressure, and weight. There are many things we can do to sharpen our memory, like getting regular exercise and eating a healthy diet. Most people can reduce their risk for Alzheimer's disease by exercising regularly and eating fewer refined carbohydrates.[11] Obesity in midlife, particularly significant belly fat, is the greatest risk for developing dementia in late life. Dementia poses both a personal and cultural threat, depending on one's perspective. However, faith leaders are increasingly stepping forward to address the dementia crisis, and families experiencing dementia are turning to clergy for support. Alzheimer's disease and related neurological disorders are the only disease forms on the rise without a cure.

---

10. Greg O'Brien, "Rocks in My Head," in Everman et al., *Dementia-Friendly Worship*, 51–62; specific page number unavailable.

11. Harvard Health Publishing and Marshall, *Alzheimer's Disease*, 17.

VIEWING DEMENTIA FROM A THEOLOGICAL PERSPECTIVE

From a theological standpoint, Christians have a responsibility to advocate for those who cannot advocate for themselves and protect vulnerable seniors with dementia. Dementia threatens the loss of self-identity, which is particularly significant in an individualistic culture. However, it is important to remember that our heavenly Father remembers and values everyone, regardless of their cognitive abilities. People with dementia can still maintain their sense of personhood, and strategies for brain health and respite care should be explored.

Despite the limitations imposed by dementia, a person's essence resides in their soul, which remains alive and receptive to ministry and friendship. This perspective is crucial for Christians who seek to serve the "least of these" and work in this field. It is essential to reject any notion that seniors with dementia are somehow lesser individuals due to their cognitive and mental losses.

We can find solace in the Lord's admonition to Joshua before entering a new phase of life: "Be strong and of good courage, be not frightened, neither be dismayed, for the Lord your God is with you wherever you go" (Josh 1:9 RSV). I reflect on my (Mike's) own experience as a caregiver for my quadriplegic son, who reminded me that the Bible contains over 365 verses urging us not to fear or worry, but to learn to trust that God is always with us.

Churches are increasingly assisting dementia caregivers, and individuals diagnosed with Alzheimer's disease and their family members should strive to stay involved in church activities for as long as possible. Some faith communities around the globe and the US are at the forefront of addressing dementia-related challenges, even if a particular church may not provide support services. Seniors with dementia can find new and creative ways to participate in church, such as illuminating others about the disease, engaging in worship, or singing in the choir. Everman et al.'s much-needed book, *Dementia-Friendly Worship*, offers outstanding, practical advice on creating worship experiences that are well suited to people with dementia. Dual choir programs, where caregivers and dementia sufferers sing together, allow for greater openness, discussion of challenges, and insights into the unique journey of those with dementia. One of our center's partners, Daphne Johnston has developed a highly portable, award-winning, dementia respite program for family caregivers (see appendix G).

For elderly Christians and those with dementia, active participation in exercise groups (e.g., balance related or social forms like tai chi), small Bible study groups, Sunday School classes, and prayer breakfasts should be embraced as health-enhancing activities that churches should promote. Caregivers report that regular, warm, and friendly conversations and a joyful countenance play a significant role in predicting healthy communication, which is especially important for people with dementia, who may experience a lack of relationships.

IMPORTANCE OF SOCIAL AND CREATIVE ACTIVITIES

The convoy model of social relations emphasizes the influence of social relationships on health and well-being.[12] It highlights the importance of individual development, lifespan perspective, and situational experiences. Social networks, support, and satisfaction are integral components of the convoy model. I (Mike) have benefited greatly from convoys of friends at play, work, and church. The emerging field of interpersonal neurobiology focuses on the neuroscience of relationships and how they positively impact the brain's plasticity, a good indication of neurological health. Enriching environments with supportive relationships, creativity, mental and physical exercise, and novel experiences have beneficial effects on the brains of the elderly, promoting resiliency and well-being.

Creative arts can also have a profound impact on individuals with dementia. An art therapist helped Lester Potts, a senior with dementia, develop his artistic skills as a watercolor painter. Potts painted over four hundred cheerful watercolor paintings that have gained recognition worldwide. His final painting depicted a black-and-white antique saw without handles, symbolizing what dementia had done to him. After Potts's passing, I (Mike) discovered an antique saw in my grandmother's basement and, guided by the Holy Spirit, gave it to Potts's son as a representation of his father's restored soul in heaven ... the handles were back on. The creative legacy left by Potts and the impact of his faith were honored by his pastor at his funeral. For more information on art therapy and other innovative programs for people with dementia, refer to appendix E, "Cognitive Dynamics."

---

12. Ajrouch et al., "Convoys of Social Relations."

ASSESSMENT

If you think you or a family member has dementia, the first step is to request an assessment of the situation from your geriatrician, primary care physician, or a local neurologist. They can help to secure an accurate diagnosis and develop a treatment plan. Dementia is diagnosed by ruling out other physical illnesses that may be causing the symptoms. Because it affects many aspects of functioning, a good assessment of dementia is conducted most thoroughly by a multidisciplinary team. This usually includes a social and medical history, a physical exam, a spiritual assessment, appropriate laboratory work, mental status exam, environmental assessment, and assessment of functional status.[13] Such an assessment is necessary to rule out other illnesses and to track the path and trajectory of the illness and the effects of care. Memory clinics and Alzheimer's disease assistance centers, which are now available in some communities, often employ multidisciplinary, geriatric teams that include the disciplines of medicine, nursing, chaplaincy, and social work. If a dementia specialist or geriatric-trained internist or family practitioner is not available, you or your family may need to involve other professionals (geriatric psychiatrists, nurses, nutritionists, geriatric-trained chaplains, social workers, physical and occupational therapists) in completing the assessment process.

When assessing dementia in a family member, determining the current stage of the disease is an important step. While there is some debate regarding whether to disclose the diagnosis to the person with dementia, it is generally recommended to share the diagnosis, as it affirms their right to know and enables early and better treatment. Identifying the primary caregiver during the assessment process is crucial. In early-stage dementia, it is beneficial to have at least one person close to the individual take on the role of primary caregiver. This involves encouraging the active involvement of other interested parties while defining roles and resolving conflicts through the assistance of nurses, chaplains, and social workers.

INTERVENTIONS

Caregivers of persons with dementia require social and psychological assistance to address various aspects such as support, long-term care planning, legal issues, family dynamics, work and financial concerns, spiritual needs,

---

13. See www.beageready.com; Parker et al., "Life Space Approach."

grief counseling, emotional support, and practical assistance in obtaining health and social services. Understanding the emotional concerns of individuals with dementia and their caregivers is essential to guide intervention efforts. Support groups or counseling may be beneficial depending on the individual's needs.

Dementia profoundly impacts functional abilities, language and speech, motor skills, judgment, reasoning, and other areas of functioning. Functional status measures can be used to assess activities of daily living, from basic tasks like bathing and toileting to higher-level activities such as managing money and driving. Environmental adaptations can be made in the early stages to compensate for memory loss. Communication strategies can be learned to assist with language and speech impairments in middle stages. As the disease progresses, the focus may shift to helping individuals cope with physical losses through home care, adult day care, or nursing home services.

Psychological impairments can occur at all stages of dementia, including depression and anxiety in the early stages and psychotic symptoms and agitation in later stages. Pharmacological treatment may be considered, but the use of psychotropic medications must be carefully monitored due to potential complications. Behavioral symptoms often result from environmental factors or inadequate pain management, so a thorough assessment of the environment and physical comfort is crucial. Non-pharmacological approaches should be prioritized for psychological problems in persons with dementia to minimize the adverse effects of medication. Collaborating with psychiatrists familiar with dementia treatment is recommended for family caregivers.

Fortunately, there are intervention strategies available to slow the progression of dementia and alleviate some of its negative effects. Several drugs on the market have shown promise in slowing the course of dementia in certain individuals. To learn about pharmacological treatment options, it is advisable to consult a local pharmacist or the doctor responsible for the family member's care for a list of alternative medications and their potential side effects. However, it's important to stay updated with the latest information on medications by reviewing the results of recent clinical drug trials. Ask a professional.[14]

14. Plans are in place to eliminate an outdated policy limiting the number of PET scans a patient can receive—a big win on an important issue to those with Alzheimer's disease. Promising new clinical trial results are in on Donanemab, a new drug to slow the progression of Alzheimer's, which will soon provide patients with more choices

To emphasize again, social isolation is a common consequence for individuals with dementia. Churches and denominations have made significant strides in involving dementia sufferers in faith-based activities for as long as possible. Encouraging their participation in worship, choir, and other programs is crucial. Churches can update congregations on new treatments through expert speakers who can translate the latest science. As the disease progresses, these communication impairments worsen, making it increasingly challenging to understand the person's intentions. Even close family caregivers may feel frustrated and become angry or short tempered when trying to communicate with the individual. Consequently, caregivers often feel ashamed to bring the person out in public or have visitors. Visitors themselves may struggle to interact with the person with dementia, resulting in unsatisfying visits. Remember, when visiting or caring for someone who has dementia, even when s/he no longer knows your name, s/he can recognize and appreciate a joyful, cheerful countenance.

PRACTICAL ASPECTS OF CARE

In addition to the social aspects, there are practical considerations in the care of individuals with dementia. In the early stages of the disease, practical strategies include assisting the person with memory aids to mitigate forgetfulness and maintain their orientation to time, person, and place. This stage is also an opportune time for future planning, which may involve establishing health care proxies and advance directives, making wills, and arranging finances for the later stages of the disease. Social workers often play a role in helping individuals with dementia and their family caregivers navigate the complexities of Medicaid, Medicare, and other health and social service programs. They can provide guidance on various support systems such as home heating assistance and food stamps that address the needs of low-income people with dementia. In the later stages of the disease, assessing informal support services and providing information about formal community supports like day care and home care can reassure caregivers that help is available and offer them respite from caregiving responsibilities.

---

for treatment. A first-of-its-kind study was released examining how hearing aids slow the progression of Alzheimer's (Harvard Health Publishing and Marshall, *Alzheimer's Disease*, 38). The CHANGE Act, which encourages early assessment and diagnosis of Alzheimer's, was introduced in Congress.

Cognitive stimulation programs can be effective with reminiscence, although their efficacy for individuals with dementia is limited. Reviews by experts in the field provide insights into the evidence surrounding these approaches. More recent programs have focused on cognitive deficits such as episodic memory, language, and numerical skills. External cognitive aids, such as organizing items used daily, medication organizers, labels, and color coding, can also enhance memory.

Apathy and lack of engagement are significant challenges for individuals with dementia, particularly in the middle and late stages of the disease, and these issues can be distressing for family caregivers. Memory albums and memory charts can be valuable tools for stimulating reminiscence, life review, and engagement, particularly in individuals with limited language abilities. Memory albums are small photo albums containing pictures of significant people, places, and events from the distant past, accompanied by simple descriptive words. Similarly, memory charts are larger boards with photographs and simple words in different panels, which can be placed in areas where the person with dementia spends time. Memory albums and memory charts are particularly effective in engaging individuals with moderate to severe dementia. Remedial intervention strategies address emotional and psychological problems as well as personality changes commonly observed in the early and middle stages of dementia. Agitation and behavioral problems are frequently encountered in the moderate to moderately severe stages. Emotional and psychological issues like depression, anxiety, delusions, and hallucinations (more prevalent in later-stage dementia) can sometimes be effectively treated with psychotropic medications, but support and reassurance also play a significant role in their management.

Behavioral analysis is often used to address agitation and behavior problems in individuals with dementia. Caregivers can play the role of behavior detectives, identifying when problematic behaviors occur and examining their antecedents and consequences. By understanding the underlying needs that are not being met, caregivers can modify the environment to restore comfort for individuals with dementia. Simple strategies like adjusting room temperature, engaging individuals in activities, reducing noise or excessive stimulation, providing reassurance, and attending to positive behaviors can help reduce behavior problems.

It is important to consider that some agitated behaviors and behavior problems may be caused by physical factors, such as pain. Therefore, before implementing behavioral intervention programs, a thorough review of potential physical causes, like arthritis pain, should be conducted. Various resources, including books and articles, provide specific guidance on handling specific behavior problems like apathy, combativeness, food refusal, insomnia, resistance to care, and wandering.[15]

While addressing agitation, behavior problems, and memory and communication decline, it is crucial not to neglect support strategies. We must remember that support for the Alzheimer's person will be different than support for the primary caregiver. Caregiving will be addressed in more detail in the chapter on caregiving. Also please note Daphne Johnston's award-winning program detailed in appendix G. Family members have a significant role in supporting individuals with dementia and their primary caregivers throughout the progression of the disease. Support can include affirming the coping abilities of persons with dementia and their caregivers in the early stages, providing reassurance and gentle touch in later stages, and implementing strategies to engage and stimulate their remaining long-term memories and language abilities. Supportive interventions also involve educating caregivers and persons with dementia about the stages of the disorder, keeping them informed about new developments in care, assisting them in accessing necessary services and resources, and helping them plan. Family care planning and problem-solving meetings, supportive counseling and reassurance, and assistance with community and institutional care options are examples of supportive interventions for family members and caregivers as dementia progresses.

HELP FOR CAREGIVERS AND OTHER FAMILY MEMBERS

Caregivers frequently experience social isolation as they devote more time around the clock to ensuring the safety of the person with dementia. Therefore, it is vital for friends and family to actively encourage caregivers to take care of themselves. Church-based respite programs for dementia family caregivers are becoming more prevalent, both in the United States and in other countries like Scotland.[16]

While religious and spiritual issues are often overlooked by professionals working with older adults, it is widely recognized that religious beliefs hold significant importance in the lives of most older adults in the United States. Many families confronted with the effects of dementia find

15. See appendix E, "Cognitive Dynamics."
16. See appendix I, "Faith in Older People."

solace in their spiritual beliefs and the support they receive from their faith communities. Prayer is often the primary coping mechanism for caregivers dealing with the demands of caregiving. Religious beliefs are particularly strong among elderly women and certain minority groups in North America.[17] Renewed contact with clergy or formal religious organizations such as churches or synagogues can provide much-needed support. Religion and spirituality can help individuals come to terms with the illness; find meaning in their lives; and make peace with family, friends, or those with whom they may have had strained relationships. Families can assist older individuals with mild dementia by incorporating spirituality and religion in life review, reminiscence, and legacy work, which helps them make sense of their experiences and find purpose. It can also involve helping persons with dementia articulate and record their preferences for medical care and funeral arrangements that align with their religious and spiritual values. Loved ones must recognize that understanding, accepting, and coming to terms with the impact of dementia on a family member can be a lengthy and gradual process, which can vary significantly among individual family members.

Family caregivers face not only the long-term responsibility of providing care but also the emotional challenge of adjusting to the gradual loss of their loved one and changing expectations within the relationship as dementia progresses. Clergy can play a crucial role in helping the entire family system cope with these emotional adjustments. They can also facilitate collaborative planning and management of care as the symptoms of dementia advance. Geriatric care managers can provide valuable support in helping families keep the person with dementia at home for as long as possible, ensuring their safety and comfort. However, when the care needs become overwhelming, the caregiver's role may include arranging for placement in a more appropriate environment like assisted living or a specialized memory care unit.

A MUCH-NEEDED GLOBAL ALLIANCE FOR BRAIN HEALTH AND MENTAL FITNESS

Jerry Wiles has helped to spearhead a comprehensive, faith-based alliance of professionals and practitioners who aim to do a better job as believers to help churches and family caregivers address brain health, including mental

---

17. Pew Forum on Religion and Public Life, *Religious Beliefs and Practices*, 29.

fitness, and various aspects of memory.[18] Wiles, with the help of others in the alliance, hopes to:

- Increase public awareness of the needs and opportunities in these areas, using various multimedia platforms
- Help create regional databases of professionals, institutions, associations, resources, and solutions addressing these issues
- Equip individuals, families, churches, and others to care for and assist those facing these challenges more effectively
- Assist churches in forming memory support groups, memory cafes, and teams of volunteers for outreach and service
- Identify, as well as produce, biblically based instructional materials addressing these and related issues
- Provide training workshops, coaching, and mentoring volunteers to recognize kingdom advancing opportunities while serving others
- Facilitate networking and collaboration among the global community of learning and practice
- Host or sponsor conferences, summits, and consultations to educate and equip wholistic disciple makers
- Facilitate the formation of a prayer network for focused intercession and connecting with other prayer ministries

A better understanding of these issues will also enhance the ability of believers of all ages in sharing the gospel and making disciples. It's not about how much education someone has but how much we remember that matters most. We can live out only what we remember.

We are grateful for his leadership and the ad hoc steering committee and advisory council giving input and direction to this initiative. Our center will support the expansion of the alliance by adding more levels of leadership and structure. Jerry and his team welcome all suggestions, connections, and input. If you are interested in being involved in some capacity, please get in touch with Dr. Jerry Wiles through the James Houston Center.

---

18. See https://www.jameshoustoncenter.com/jerry-wiles.

CONCLUSION

Dementia presents major challenges because it affects emotional, physical, mental, social, and spiritual functioning. Coping with Alzheimer's disease is demanding on the dementia sufferer and his/her family. Family caregivers play a critical role in the care of a family member with Alzheimer's disease, whether at home or in an institutional setting. An interdisciplinary, wholistic, comprehensive approach by all is best, because the disease affects the bio-psycho-social-spiritual aspects of life during all phases of care. Christians have a special opportunity to develop respite programs to help families cope with collapse.

DEMENTIA AND EXERCISE

Exercise boosts brain connections, generates new brain cells, and reduces inflammation. Exercise increases the hormone klotho, a marker for longevity, and protects against cognitive decline (levels can increase after 20 minutes of vigorous exercise). Regular aerobic activity (150 minutes per week of moderate intensity activity such as brisk walking) significantly reduces the risk of cardiovascular disease, type 2 DM, hyperlipidemia, HTN, anxiety, depression, and obesity, which are all risk factors for cognitive decline. In one study, daily brisk walks led to a 40 percent lower risk of developing Alzheimer's or another dementia in later life (only 15 minutes a day may be effective). Leg strength is correlated with better cognitive function.[19] Physical activities increase the synthesis of brain-derived neurotrophic factor (BDNF), which acts as a "neuron fertilizer." The importance of unwinding and restoration for brain health are also well accepted by most neurologists.[20]

SWIMMING IS A CLEAN-BRAIN, HEALTH-ENHANCING STRATEGY

Most mornings you will find me (Mike) at the University of Alabama's outdoor pool. Most of the swimmers are very positive-minded friends and acquaintances, and I look forward to seeing them. Some are members of my convoy of friends who are aging in time with me. Though it can be a

---

19. Harvard Health Publishing and Marshall, *Alzheimer's Disease*, 17.
20. Harvard Health Publishing and Marshall, *Alzheimer's Disease*, 18–19.

cold entry in the winter months, just like other forms of exercise on land, swimming and water aerobics are some of the best exercises available to most aging folks. Bartlett Hess was founder of the Evangelical Presbyterian denomination. He became my pastor during my postdoctoral study at the University of Michigan. He was the perfect pastor for me at that time. He was a regular swimmer in the aquatic facilities at the University of Michigan. He was a remarkable man, with doctoral degrees in theology and history, and he became one of my good friends while I was completing my postdoc. He was a good example of someone aging successfully.[21] He understood that forms of water-based exercise improve cardio fitness, build strength, elevate mood, ease joint pain, help with sleeping better, and reduce your risk for heart disease, diabetes, dementia, and cancer. Pretty good outcomes for an investment of few hours a week.

When your body becomes buoyant in the water, good things happen! Your joints experience less impact—welcome information to those suffering from arthritis, which affects about 70 percent of older Americans. Certain forms of exercise are doable in an aquatic environment (like squats). Movements in the water are often smooth and flowing, so water activities are less likely to aggravate injuries. Movement in the water is slowed and less likely to aggravate existing injuries. Jogging and other forms of exercise in the water provide more resistance, so they burn more calories and are good for cardio and strength exercises.[22]

DEMENTIA AND NUTRITION

Most are not aware that obesity in midlife increases the risk of dementia by 40 percent. Individuals who spend more time watching TV have a greater risk of Alzheimer's. More complex activities provide greater protection. The best idea is to find something that keeps you active, challenges your brain, and makes you happy. Elliptical machines and recumbent bikes are good on the joints. Tai chi, ballroom dancing, and swimming, as noted, are helpful. The number of hours individuals sit per day is a much better predictor of future cognitive decline than their daily exercise regimen.

---

21. Founding five churches of over five thousand members each, he demonstrated the efficacy of small groups to church growth and life.

22. Harvard Health Publishing, "Advantages of Water-Based Exercise."

Extended periods of sedentary behavior negate the benefits of twenty to thirty minutes of exercise.[23]

DIET AND NUTRITION

There is evidence that a plant-based diet is associated with a 28-percent lower risk of dementia, while those who consume meat have twice the risk of developing dementia. Processed foods high in sugar and saturated fats are toxic to the brain, and excessive sugar consumption is linked to brain atrophy. Sugar is considered a significant contributor to Alzheimer's development, causing cellular stress, insulin resistance, neuronal starvation, impaired communication, inflammation, and sticky amyloid buildup. Stevia is often recommended as a safe sweetener.[24]

Midlife high cholesterol increases the risk of Alzheimer's by over 50 percent. In a women's health study at Harvard, women with the highest saturated fat intake had a 65-percent higher risk of brain dysfunction.[25] Omega-3 fatty acids are beneficial for the brain and can be obtained from sources such as wild fish, walnuts, chia seeds, flaxseed, hempseed, and green leafy vegetables like kale and spinach. Extra-virgin olive oil is preferred over coconut oil. For brain-healthy snacks, opt for fruits, vegetables, hummus, bean dips, purees, whole wheat bread, green tea, coffee, nuts, and seeds. On the other hand, it's best to avoid processed foods, processed sweets, sugary drinks, and excessive alcohol.

The MIND diet, a combination of the Mediterranean and DASH diets, has been developed at Rush University. Strict adherence to this diet has been shown to reduce Alzheimer's risk by 50 percent. It emphasizes high vegetable consumption and a favorable ratio of unsaturated to saturated fats.[26]

---

23. Harvard Health Publishing and Marshall, *Alzheimer's Disease*, 17.
24. Harvard Health Publishing and Marshall, *Alzheimer's Disease*, 18.
25. Health & Nutrition Letter, "Fat Choices," para. 4; see also Harvard Health Publishing, "Protect Your Brain."
26. Harvard Health Publishing and Marshall, *Alzheimer's Disease*, 18.

IV. Our Selves in Community

Chapter 11

A Christian's Caregiving Ministry

CHRISTIAN MINISTRY IS WHEREVER YOU ARE, FOR AS LONG AS YOU LIVE!

My (Jim's) ministry is now in a seniors' home for assisted living. One of my daughters, Claire, is a flight attendant on an airline. She could have retired several years ago, but she is called to minister more than to having a job. My son is a management consultant, but in retirement, he writes books on business ethics in secular language, but with a Christian motive. Another daughter adores being a Christian grandmother for many grandchildren, while yet another daughter does a ministry of overseas charity to peasant women, within her husband's business. For me, it is my crown and joy to have all my children serving the Lord in such a variety of ways.

THE REFORMED DOCTRINE OF THE PRIESTHOOD OF ALL BELIEVERS

The words of God to the Israelites, "You shall be to me a kingdom of priests and a holy nation" (Exod 19:6 NKJV), are applied in the New Testament to the church of God (1 Pet 2:5, 9; 5:10; Rev 1:6; 5:10; 20:6). This was upheld by the early fathers, such as Tertullian and Hippolytus. Only as the church became more institutionalized did this biblical doctrine get lost. It was recovered in the Reformation, only to be lost again, even until now. Only now are small house churches seeking to recover this primitive practice of seeing themselves as God's priests, wherever they are and whatever they do.

When we founded Regent College, ca. 1968–70, we sought to recover the priesthood of all believers, as well as the identity of being "mere Christians." C. S. Lewis recovered this theme from Richard Baxter after the Civil War of the mid-seventeenth century. I recall that Lewis was often asked what kind of Anglican he was. Lewis's laconic reply was "A man of the foothills, never very high, nor very low."

BE A GOOD CHRISTIAN WHEREVER YOU ARE AND IN WHATEVER LINE OF WORK YOU CHOOSE

I shocked a conference of some two hundred pastors in Hong Kong, some years ago, by charging them with Buddhist practice! For a seriously committed Buddhist will clothe himself in the saffron robes of a monk, by his serious commitment! After the meeting, an alumnus showed me my correspondence with him, years before. As a serious Christian, I dissuaded him as a government auditor from leaving his profession, and even from going to Regent's summer school. Rather, he should go to Oxford University, to its summer school in public administration, to improve his professional calling. Eventually, he became the public auditor of Hong Kong. Likewise, a Canadian student shared that he had two loves: being a pastor and being a director of drama. I told him we had few Christian dramatists and lots of pastors. Strategically, he should be a Christian dramatist, which he still is!

Now that I am in a seniors' home for assisted living, I have a new ministry. Like the apostle Paul, even if we feel imprisoned by our circumstances, we can serve the Lord. When I was a small boy, recovering from severe illness, I heard of another small boy crippled in bed. He served the Lord by writing Scripture texts, tied to a string, to be picked up by passersby! Eighty years later, the story still moves me!

The apostle Paul testified that whatever state he was in, he could serve the Lord. He found ways to serve the Lord in prison, wearily traveling the long Roman roads, as a tentmaker, and even in a storm at sea and in a shipwreck. As he confides to the Corinthian Christians, he served the Lord through much affliction and bodily suffering, and in having permanently "a thorn in the flesh" (2 Cor 12:7 NKJV). "For when I am weak, then I am strong" (2 Cor 12:10 NKJV). Even when he thought he was making a fool of himself before others, his ministry continued! Such divine wisdom given to him is also indomitable courage!

We, too, embody our ministry by the environment in which God has placed us. No matter what our circumstances may be, whether we are in church, in the street, or in our invalid bedroom, we can serve the Lord. Too often, we are brainwashed to assume it is only the pastors who have a Christian ministry. What a tragic loss of Christian ministerial potential for the kingdom of God. One need go no further than to examine the worldwide ministry of Joni Eareckson, quadriplegic for most of her life.[1] Her worldwide ministry and advocacy for people with physical limitations makes anyone who knows her want to bury the word *disabled*. As busy as she is, she wrote our (Mike) quadriplegic son a beautiful, yet honest, encouraging letter that the entire family, including Mike, will treasure for our remaining time in this world.

I (Jim) recently received an email from a Christian friend and publisher in China who has spent many years under house arrest. In three shifts every twenty-four hours, he is being watched, while he continues to translate English Christian books and to print them for publication in China. Like the apostle Paul, he truly has his "prison ministry," undaunted and in perseverance, serving the Lord. Bedridden, restricted physically, wherever we are, we are called to serve the Lord, until our dying breath!

LATE-LIFE PURPOSE

Pray to our heavenly Father to learn his late-life purpose for you, and perhaps you will discover, as Jim Houston has, that your purpose is right where you live! Or as Jim has advised so many at Regent and all over the world, serve the Lord in your current profession, but with a primary Christian identity. And I (Mike) appeal to you, do not make the same mistake our ageist culture continues to make. There is no one in the world just like you, so you have the capacity for a unique ministry no matter what your age. Come join our army of senior saints, not perfect, but certainly not limited by your age, in the Holy Spirit–empowered ministry God has given you!

---

1. See https://joniandfriends.org/.

Chapter 12

Caregiving for Aging Parents and Loved Ones

When Jesus saw his mother, and the disciple whom he loved standing near, he said to his mother, "Woman, behold, your son!" Then he said to the disciple, "Behold, your mother!" And from that hour the disciple took her to his own home.
(John 19:26–27 RSV)

REGARDLESS OF ONE'S RELIGIOUS beliefs, the example set by Jesus in caring for his mother during his crucifixion inspires us all to evaluate our own plans for caring for aging parents and loved ones. Personally, I (Mike) had little knowledge about caregiving when my father required my assistance, and being stationed overseas made it even more challenging. I was also unprepared for caregiving when my older son experienced a spinal cord injury. However, Jim's devoted care for his wife has served as an exemplary model for me and others involved in family caregiving.

Jim and I have worked diligently to share our own experiences with aging, as well as our research on parent care, in the development of an evidence-based parent care program called the AgeReady program. Initially implemented for military families, we later extended its reach to congregations and employees of large organizations. This program assists older individuals in preparing for a longer life and helps them prepare to care for their aging parents and loved ones.

Conversations among mid-lifers often gravitate toward the challenges of caring for aging parents. Unfortunately, our research reveals that many people are unprepared to provide such care. I, for example, was wholly unprepared when my father fell ill and passed away while I was serving in the first Iraq war. This personal experience fueled my drive to create a parent care program. It began during my military service when the Army Medical Department approved my assignment to a two-year, National Institute on Aging postdoctoral fellowship at the University of Michigan, as described in a separate chapter.

I learned after my father's death that a bus tour from his aging-in-place facility took a tour of lovely homes in my dad's hometown. Several on that tour told me of his reaction when they had passed the home he had built for his family. With tears rolling down his cheek, he had managed to get out the words, "That's my home." My sister and I had rushed the decision of moving him to the aging-in-place facility. It taught me the importance of "details." Later, my brother-in-law told me that he thought Dad had starved himself to death.

Returning to the story of Jesus, we witness his decision to entrust the care of his mother to John, one of his disciples and possibly his closest friend. While we do not know the full reasons behind Jesus's decision, honoring one's father and mother is a recurring theme in the teachings of various world religions. Jesus, through his own example on the cross, affirmed the significance of caring for parents. The apostle Paul reiterated the importance of parental caregiving, emphasizing the often-overlooked benefits that come to those who fulfill their responsibilities toward their parents (1 Tim 5:4–8).

Despite the consistency of these instructions across different religions, most churches, synagogues, mosques, and other faith communities in the United States do not offer practical guidance on parent care for adult children and their older family members. While breakthroughs are being made in areas like dementia care, as detailed in this book's appendices, this situation partly stems from the general lack of applied gerontological research and training within faith-based communities. Consequently, conscientious religious leaders, both professional and lay, find themselves ill equipped to address the growing needs of older individuals within their faith communities and families.[1]

However, faith communities are well positioned to assist American families in planning for the care of their older members. Americans hold strong religious beliefs and regularly attend religious services, often relying on their faith and the counsel of clergy when faced with family issues, rather

---

1. Parker et al., "Parent Care and Religion."

than turning to social services or other community agencies. This reliance on faith and clergy is particularly evident among underserved groups. Furthermore, research indicates a positive correlation between faith, religious attendance, and good health, especially in later years. We believe that now is the opportune time for churches to help individuals plan for caregiving and for longer lives.

In this chapter we address faith-based parent care readiness and training in four ways. *First*, we provide a brief overview of the relevant literature on parent care. *Next*, we connect an empirically based theoretical model of successful aging, which incorporates spirituality, to parent care assessment and planning. Leaders in faith communities can employ this conceptual model to develop comprehensive parent care training programs for their congregations. *Third*, we propose a community-based framework that has been empirically tested and incorporates a faith-sensitive, ecumenical approach to parent care training. The aim of this framework is to enhance the well-being of older individuals. *Additionally*, we adapt an evidence-based parent care intervention program, informed by previous research sponsored by the Hartford Foundation and the Gerontological Society of America at the U.S. Air War College, specifically tailored for faith-based communities. Our goal is to provide religious leaders and human service providers interested in faith-based work with an effective approach to prepare families for the developmental task and religious duty of "honoring mother and father."[2]

AN OVERVIEW OF PARENT CARE IN THE US

The United States has witnessed several significant societal changes, including increased life expectancy, greater female participation in the labor force, declining fertility rates, expanded family mobility and geographic separation, and the development of diverse multigenerational family structures. These changes have had an impact on families, including those within faith communities, and their ability to care for older family members. Research on family caregiving suggests that both those providing care in close proximity and those providing care from a distance are ill prepared for the normative developmental task of caring for older family members. Many individuals find themselves reacting to health care crises faced by their elderly family members rather than being proactive in their

2. Parker et al., "Parent Care and Religion."

caregiving role. As the population continues to age, caregiving responsibilities have become increasingly important, especially with older persons, whether living at home or in community settings, who require assistance due to chronic disease and disability.

Employers and service organizations have become increasingly aware of the potential negative impact of parent care on productivity. Although the costs of caregiving to religious organizations have not been extensively studied, such as the impact on members' ability to donate time and money due to caregiving responsibilities, parent care does impose costs on both employers and employees. A national study estimated that the costs associated with replacing employees, absenteeism, workday interruptions, eldercare crises, and supervisors' time amounted to an aggregate cost of billions of dollars due to decreased productivity resulting from caregiving responsibilities. The economic value of informal family caregiving has been estimated to be about $600 billion annually.[3] Perhaps you have experienced conflicting commitments involving your work, family obligations, and caregiving duties for one or more of your parents or in-laws.

Despite the availability of numerous books, journal articles, and internet sites to assist people faced with filial responsibilities, there is a lack of thorough investigation into the effects and potential benefits of these informational sources. Many families dealing with a parent care crisis do not use this information. For those who do access it, the information is often presented in a complex and confusing manner. Caregivers often try to navigate extensive nonessential information in search of answers to their specific questions without the guidance and support of experts.

A growing number of studies have focused on caregiving interventions.[4] Literature reviews indicate that participating in individual and group intervention programs for caregivers, as well as utilizing day care and other community resources for care recipients, can effectively support family caregivers in maintaining cognitively and physically impaired older individuals in community settings. In fact, there are now studies suggesting that caregiver support programs can delay nursing home placement and reduce health care costs for care recipients. The findings indicating changes of only some variables align with the conclusions of many review studies, which suggest that caregiver support groups tend to have small to moderate effects on caregiver outcomes. While caregivers generally express high

---

3. Reinhard et al., "Valuing the Invaluable 2023," para. 1.
4. Roff et al., "Family-Social Tasks."

satisfaction and subjective benefit from interventions, most projects find relatively small to moderate effects on outcomes related to general well-being, burden, and depression.[5]

Preliminary research conducted with one of the largest employers of individuals who live far away from their parents, the US military, suggests that a lack of preparedness for parent care places senior-ranking military members at higher risk for vocational, family, and health-related problems. Officer satisfaction with a parent care plan was found to be inversely related to officer worry, even when accounting for various other variables in a structural equation model. This research provides robust, quantitative support to previous qualitative findings by other researchers regarding long-distance caregiving and further indicates that officer satisfaction with a realistic parent care plan reduces worry among officers about their parents.[6]

The finding that satisfaction with parents' future plans significantly reduces adult children's worry about their parents' well-being underscores the importance of parents' making and discussing future plans with their children. Preliminary research suggests that only 8 to 17 percent of the population actively plan for their end of life care by having conversations with their children about their wishes and completing an advance directive. Concerns about burdening their children and difficulties in coping with the uncertainties of dying or end of life care often lead parents to avoid making plans or discussing them with their children.

Moreover, the prospect of losing a parent is traumatic for most children, and initiating a conversation about end of life plans becomes challenging when a parent insists that such plans are unnecessary. When families lack a sense of what should be included in a plan or when there are existing parent-child relationship issues, adult children often encounter resistance from their aging parents when trying to develop a plan. However, an effective presentation of the parent care planning process can provide adult children with an opportunity to engage their parents in this crucial yet difficult topic. This process allows parents to express their wishes and preferences regarding medical, legal, environmental, and emotional aspects before the onset of diseases and disabilities that may render them unable to make decisions for themselves.

Both adult children and their parents require encouragement and support to actively participate in the creation of an individualized family

5. Parker et al., "Parent Care and Religion."
6. Roff et al., "Family-Social Tasks," 29.

plan. Unfortunately, many adult children lack the motivation to engage in parent care training when their parents are still healthy. This is unfortunate, because most tasks associated with proactive parent care planning are best completed when parents can fully participate in the process. Some parent care tasks even require the parents' full understanding, involvement, and approval.

Clergy and other pastoral professionals possess unique qualifications to reinforce the importance of proactive parent care preparation. Just as ministers have advocated for premarital counseling, religious leaders can use their moral authority and religious teachings to underscore the need for families to prepare for the developmental responsibility of parent care. Adult children, spouses, and other family and nonfamily caregivers within faith-based communities can also play crucial roles in maintaining the health and independence of older individuals. To address these issues effectively, religious leaders need proper training and access to proven resources and methods to develop and promote exemplary programs.

Recent polls have found that 95 percent of Americans aged fifty or older believe in God, and 42 to 46 percent of Americans of all ages have attended religious services within the past seven days.[7] While religious involvement in America appears to be strong,[8] there is often a significant disconnect between faith-based communities and professional and academic organizations. This lack of connection hinders the development and evaluation of essential eldercare programs within faith-based communities. One of the barriers to realizing the potential of faith-based approaches in addressing people's needs, such as parent care training, is the resistance from professional and academic organizations to recognize and appreciate the value of spirituality and partnerships with faith-based organizations. Interestingly, for most of recorded history, religion and health professions like medicine, social work, and nursing were closely intertwined, with the past two centuries witnessing a separation. It was only toward the end of the twentieth century that scientific exploration of the intersection of religion, spirituality, health, and aging began.[9]

In recent years, scientists and health care professionals from various disciplines have increasingly acknowledged the strong and positive

---

7. For current figures, see https://www.pewresearch.org/religious-landscape-study/database/.

8. Koenig, "83-Year-Old Woman."

9. Crowther et al., "Rowe and Kahn's Model."

relationship between faith and health, stimulating interest in collaborations between professionals and faith-based organizations. Notably, the Joint Commission on Accreditation of Healthcare Organizations, almost three quarters of US medical schools, and several other professional educational programs and organizations now provide instruction and guidelines on assessing spirituality and incorporating it into clinical care. The work of the now-deceased Dave Larson and currently the work of Harold Koenig and others have shed light on the general neglect of spirituality by the research community in understanding various physical and mental health outcomes. Although progress has been made since Larson's initial work in the late 1980s, there is still much to be accomplished in establishing effective partnerships that address specific needs. Evidence-based theories are essential as a foundation for interventions that bridge these barriers.

A MODEL OF SUCCESSFUL, RESILIENT AGING

To promote successful aging among older individuals, adult children engaged in parent care can benefit from guidelines to support their parents' well-being. Similarly, clergy and lay leaders from faith-based communities have a responsibility to offer programs and support services to caregiving adults that meet the requirements of their roles. The primary objective of these programs should be to facilitate successful aging among older members. Programs should be grounded in theory and supported by evidence-based guidelines. The theoretical model should acknowledge the scientific importance of spirituality in successful aging. In line with the purpose of this chapter, we recommend using a model that recognizes the role of spirituality and facilitates faith-based partnerships, aligning with scientific findings.

The theoretical incorporation of spirituality into current models of successful aging represents an important acknowledgment of the research findings of the past five decades. In keeping with this expanded model, we have defined positive spirituality as a developing and internalized personal relationship with the sacred or transcendent that is not bound by gender, race, ethnicity, economics, or class, and as a dynamic that promotes the wellness and welfare of self and others.[10] The addition of positive spirituality to earlier models of successful aging bridges the gap between theory and

---

10. Crowther et al., "Rowe and Kahn's Model."

practice, especially when we seek creative solutions that include spiritual communities to address multiple problems.

Religious leaders can use this definition and the expanded model to assist adult children and their parents in understanding the interdependent biological, psychological, social, and spiritual processes associated with aging and their connections to the development of an effective parent care plan. Active engagement in life is encouraged by the model and the definition of positive spirituality, and parent care plans should foster the active involvement of older persons in the lives of their families and communities, while affirming their traditional leadership roles in religious communities.

A FRAMEWORK OF FAITH-BASED INTERVENTIONS

A third purpose of this chapter is to introduce religious leaders, adult children, aging persons, and directors of human resource departments to a proven framework and an online program called AgeReady for developing and implementing an age-friendly parent care intervention program.[11]

The AgeReady intervention program is based on a military paradigm that has been applied and tailored for use in unique congregational contexts and large organizations like universities, while including local communities as the conceptual contexts for intervention.

Faith-based communities can apply the definition of spirituality and the expanded model of successful aging (provided above) as they develop parent care training programs. Parent care ministries should address specific outcomes for the parent and the caregiving adults, including maximizing cognitive and physical fitness, avoiding disease and disability, remaining actively engaged in life, and experiencing positive spiritual growth.

Religious leaders can use our evidence-based, fourfold theoretical model (medical, spiritual-emotional, familial, and legal-financial) to help adult children and their parents understand the interdependent biological, psychological, social, and spiritual processes associated with aging and their connections to the development of an effective parent care plan. Our model and definition of positive spirituality encourage active engagement in life. Parent care plans should foster the active involvement of older persons in the lives of their families and communities, while affirming their traditional leadership roles in religious communities.

---

11. See www.beageready.com.

AGEREADY INTERVENTION PROGRAM

The fourth objective of this chapter is to present a targeted intervention program for parent care that can be implemented within faith communities, aligning with the theoretical model and framework for faith-based partnerships. This program is partially inspired by a military parent care program designed to enhance officers' preparedness in caring for their parents. In the military, all personnel with dependent family members are required to create a family care plan before deployment. This plan addresses the medical, legal, and spiritual well-being of surviving family members in case the service member—be it a soldier, sailor, airman, or marine—does not return. Recognizing the importance of caring for aging parents, I (Mike) have advocated expanding the traditional military family care plan to include provisions for the elderly parents of military personnel. Clinical studies are currently underway to modify the existing family care plan used by the US military, incorporating considerations for older and disabled loved ones. Faith-based community leaders can draw valuable insights from the experiences of military families to help their members develop family care plans that encompass the needs of older loved ones.

Under the sponsorship of the U.S. Army Medical Department, the National Institute on Aging, the John A. Hartford Foundation, and the Gerontological Society of America, I (Mike) have developed tools to aid military personnel, senior-ranking officers, their spouses, and their parents in creating a parent care plan for the future. The study aimed to assess the effectiveness of the assessment, workshop, and educational materials in helping adult children fulfill specific parent care responsibilities and enhance their readiness for present and future caregiving duties. A Parent Care Readiness Assessment (PCRA) instrument was developed to gauge the preparedness level of military personnel. The instrument was administered to fifty midlife careerists stationed at the U.S. Air War College, Maxwell Air Force Base. Using a 2x2 randomized, partial crossover design, fifty participants were randomly assigned to either the experimental group or the control group. The experimental group received a two-hour workshop covering medical, legal-financial, family-social, and spiritual-emotional tasks, along with supporting computer-accessed materials and workbook. Both groups completed the PCRA at baseline and a three-month follow-up. Preliminary findings from ongoing field trials suggest that workshop participants, along with those who received the support materials, completed more parent care tasks and exhibited higher levels of confidence about their future as caregivers compared to the control group of caregivers.

Communities of faith can adapt the Parent Care Readiness Intervention Program, originally developed for military families, to help congregational families make informed choices about parent care responsibilities.

The AgeReady Intervention Program and Planning Process

The Parent Care Readiness Program (PCRP), now AgeReady, connects leaders in communities of faith with families, providing them with resources and information related to parent care. This program offers practical guidance to help families to develop a comprehensive care plan.

The AgeReady program involves a series of specific tasks relevant to older adults' changing circumstances. The intervention should be regarded as a dynamic process that requires ongoing reassessment as the older adult's circumstances change.

The tasks involved in parent care are categorized into four domains: medical, legal-financial, family-social, and spiritual-emotional tasks. Each domain represents real-life challenges older adults are likely to face. Effective time management and problem-solving strategies recommend breaking down complex challenges into essential tasks. This approach helps people make realistic progress and prevents them from feeling overwhelmed.

The AgeReady model emphasizes the importance of assessing all four domains and beginning by completing the tasks caregivers deem to be of highest priority. The intent is to prevent information overload by information and resources for each specific task. The model recognizes that planning and completing tasks are part of an ongoing process as the functional and health status of the older adult change.

The current AgeReady program is available now online to individuals, families, and churches.[12]

The principal components of the AgeReady program include:

1. AgeReady assessment: This assessment evaluates the parent care readiness of individuals and families and provides tailored information to address their unique needs.

2. AgeReady resources for each task offer guidance and support in completing the various tasks associated with parent care.

12. See www.beageready.com, or contact our center (www.jameshoustoncenter.com).

3. AgeReady website: This online platform provides automatic internet links, resources, and information that assist caregivers in accomplishing each task.

4. Workshop curriculum: A two- or five-hour workshop, incorporating a PowerPoint presentation with selected clips from Hollywood movies and television programs, supplements the AgeReady program online and other available resources. This workshop provides an overview of medical, legal-financial, family, and spiritual tasks.

5. Individual family consultation: Local professionals such as social workers, geriatric care managers, elder law attorneys, and geriatricians offer personalized consultations as needed.

By adapting and implementing the AgeReady and intervention program within congregational families, communities of faith can equip caregivers with the necessary tools and knowledge to navigate the complexities of parent care and make conscious, informed choices.

The assessment process is a crucial feature of the parent care training program known as AgeReady.

AgeReady's readiness assessment helps families identify and prioritize the specific tasks involved in caring for their aging family members. This assessment was developed based on feedback from focus group sessions with volunteers from the U.S. Army and U.S. Air War Colleges, as well as input from professional experts in various fields. The AgeReady assessments consist of regularly updated sets of approximately ten tasks for each of the four domains.[13]

The AgeReady assessment provides caregivers with valuable information such as completion rates, indicating readiness, and a sense of task priority or importance. It also identifies tasks that could have been completed more effectively. Examples of these tasks include helping parents create a list of their health care providers, discussing the pros and cons of completing a durable power of attorney, and facilitating a family conference to develop care plans. Furthermore, the assessment highlights tasks that need to be completed and provides a sense of when they should be addressed. The AgeReady program delivers customized outcomes to caregivers and care recipients, addressing each family's unique needs and preferences.

---

13. Preliminary measures of internal consistency and task alignment by domain have shown statistically acceptable levels.

The AgeReady training program should be open to anyone interested in attending the workshop, as parent care is a responsibility that nearly everyone will face in their own life course. Certain groups are particularly prone to this task. Women, traditionally the primary caregivers, are increasingly entering the workforce, which puts them at higher risk of burden and burnout. Women, including wives, daughters, and daughters-in-law, have historically provided much of the home care for ill and disabled family members. Approximately 40 percent of women providing care for aging relatives are also simultaneously caring for children, often due to delayed childbearing and multigenerational caregiving. In general, the impact of parent care is most noticeable for adult children in midlife, as they are at a higher risk of facing crises related to their aging parents. Adult children of frail elderly individuals living in the community are particularly vulnerable to responding to health care emergencies, such as falls or strokes. Currently, we are exploring the benefits of involving parents in the training alongside their adult children, as their active participation in planning their own care may have advantages such as self-care and improved communication.

Small congregations with limited resources should consider forming partnerships with other religious groups, professional organizations, academic institutions, and subject matter experts to develop initiatives for parent care training. Denominational and other congregation-serving organizations may want to initiate AgeReady training programs for their congregations.

The involvement of local subject matter experts in the training process is highly encouraged. Their participation can enhance and support the specific content covered online. The AgeReady program also encourages the establishment of professional relationships with local geriatricians, elder law attorneys, geriatric care managers, and other relevant professionals. For maximum benefit, these experts should share similar spiritual beliefs and practices as the sponsoring organization and be familiar with both the parent care training program and the entire parent care program. The workshop materials align with the AgeReady website, app, tailored assessments, and task-specific resources to aid participants in completing each task effectively.

AgeReady introduces an intervention strategy that capitalizes on the potential of computer, internet, and app technologies. As internet technology continues to advance at a rapid pace, the accessibility to these resources may increase. Leveraging these mediums for interventions holds immense promise in significantly reducing caregiver burden for adult children who live both near and far from their aging parents, ultimately enhancing their parents' quality of life. As costs decrease and user friendliness improves, a large percentage of seniors will rely on the internet for communication and support. Interactive health communications utilizing this distribution system will play a vital role in future support services. With the implementation of BeAgeReady.com, families, church groups, and organizations (HR reps welcomed) have immediate access to resources that address their most pressing care needs, such as locating home health care or adult day care services. AgeReady facilitates the downloading of task-specific information, allowing caregivers and care recipients to quickly access critical information for a particular task. Additionally, hard copies of the information are also provided for convenience.

To encourage participation in the program, faith-based organizations can offer computer access and training as incentives. Many parents who lack computer literacy would benefit greatly from internet and web access. As part of their parent care plan, regular communication with more tech-savvy adult children and grandchildren can take place through an internet site associated with their respective church, synagogue, or mosque.

Conclusions and Implications

How can families, who are the primary caregivers of older Americans, collaborate with professionals from various health-related disciplines to address the challenges posed by the expanding aging population in the US? Specifically, how can religious leaders help prepare families for the responsibilities and religious obligations of caring for their parents and facing their own aging and longer lifespans?

While it is impossible to fully prepare for unforeseen events such as acts of terrorism, families within the military have already taken steps to minimize the long-term consequences of such traumas through intergenerational family care plans. Similarly, religious leaders can guide their congregations in being better prepared for the unexpected, such as acts of terrorism, weather disasters, auto accidents, or health crises, by proactively addressing the predictable challenges of life, including parent care. Organized religious communities are ideally positioned to emphasize the significance of parent care as a normal role, requiring proactive preparation as a religious privilege. They can ensure that faith-based programs are available to help families prepare for the developmental task of parent care and personal longevity. This program could become one of organized religions' contributions to family security.

The unifying framework and theoretical basis for this intervention, along with the demographic imperative for faith-based parent care interventions, call for a reversal in the recent trend of separating spirituality, organized religion, non-faith-based institutions, and academic and health care professionals. This program aims to prepare adult children for the developmental task of parent care, reducing caregiver anxiety and boosting confidence through the proactive completion of age-friendly caregiving tasks. By applying twenty-first-century information and service technologies, this program equips families to provide intelligent and loving care to their aging parents or other relatives. Moreover, improved readiness in caregiving allows members of faith-based organizations to maintain productive employment or engage in volunteer services and activities, while ensuring a higher quality of life for their older loved ones.

As our society grapples with the increasing costs of health care, there is a pressing need for creative solutions to address the impending health crisis. The religious community and the health care industry will need to collaborate in search of such solutions. In this context, how will the aging church respond? Our program, built upon an expanded Rowe and Kahn (1998) theory[14] and a faith-based community framework, possesses the potential to generate interest and foster collaborations across religious, denominational, racial, and class boundaries. This process can contribute to unifying faith communities around the significant task of honoring parents. In this century, both the health care industry and religious organizations will increasingly recognize the importance of the spiritual dimension in bridging the gap between medical advancements and our way of life.

14. Myers et al., "Feasibility Study."

Chapter 13

AgeReady

OVERVIEWS FOR EACH OF THE FOUR DOMAINS OF CAREGIVING TASKS

Medical Tasks

As people age, they often develop chronic conditions that require ongoing medical care. However, modern medicine tends to focus on specific medical encounters rather than on a comprehensive approach to chronic care. As a family member, it's important to understand how medical care for older adults works in the US and in your community. Good geriatric care involves a synthesis of medical and social attention to address an individual's functional status and allow them to enjoy as normal a lifestyle as possible. This requires coordination among multiple professionals and communication with family members to avoid duplication and ensure better health outcomes. It's also important to understand long-term care services and what's available in your community.

Task Name: Geriatric Assessment
Task Overview

- A comprehensive geriatric assessment is an evaluation to determine, among other things, the functional capabilities of an older adult to develop a plan for care during the aging process. This tool can improve health care outcomes for the older adult and can be beneficial to you when helping to manage their care.

- This assessment can help to ensure their concerns are accurately diagnosed and they receive the most effective treatments and preventive health care possible. If the older adult has a geriatric physician; you can schedule it with them. If not, their primary care provider should be able to complete this assessment as well.

Task Question: Have you completed a comprehensive geriatric assessment with the older adult's geriatric physician or primary care physician?

Learn More: What Is a Comprehensive Geriatric Assessment?

- This assessment is a tool used by health care practitioners to evaluate an older adult's physical and mental health to determine and optimize a plan for their care.
- The findings may indicate that plans need to be made to ensure the older adult's safety and well-being, such as making new housing arrangements or getting in-home assistance.

Benefit of a Comprehensive Geriatric Assessment

- To determine the older adult's functional status
- To help in the development of a long-term plan
- To provide context for assessing any change in future health

Preparing for the Assessment

- Prior to the assessment, a family member or caregiver should attempt to track the older adult's past and current major illnesses, conditions, and surgeries, including the information on allergies and adverse medication reactions.
- Each time they are scheduled for an evaluation, a family member or caregiver should compile a list of symptoms or complaints and should be encouraged to work with the older adult to keep this information current.
- If possible, you (or another caregiver) should attend the appointment.

What to Expect

- Psychosocial assessment
- Medication review
- Comprehensive physical exam
- Mental status exam
- Environmental assessment
- Housing adaptations and barriers
- Mobility
- Spiritual assessment
- Functional assessment
- The overall research indicated that an assessment could lead to solving problems and helping a parent remain independent longer.
- A good interdisciplinary medical care plan can result in fewer accidents or falls, less illness, a longer life, more quality of life, and greater independence.

Resources

- The Health in Aging Foundation tells consumers how to find geriatric health professionals.
- Find a geriatric health care professional.
- *The Merck Manual of Geriatrics* provides information about what occurs when a physician performs a geriatric assessment.[1]
- Comprehensive geriatric assessment

Other Medical Domain Topics

- Health care team
- Medicine management
- Evaluate driving skills
- Geriatric care manager

1. Berkow and Beers, *Merck Manual.*

- Assess facility
- Exercise and activity plan
- Cognitive impairment/dementia evaluation
- Iatrogenesis

Legal-Financial Tasks

The legal and financial issues associated with aging parents' care can be complex, but it's crucial to address them openly to avoid major problems. This includes reviewing legal and financial documents, analyzing income and benefits, assessing the parent's budget and future needs, and reviewing insurance coverage and end of life care provisions. Coordinated assistance from an elder law attorney, a financial planner, an accountant, and/or a geriatric care manager can help complete these tasks effectively.

Task Name: Legal Documents
Task Overview

- Many families and caregivers wait until a health crisis before considering a plan for the older adult's long-term care. It is important to develop and review legal documents before anything happens to represent the wishes of the older adult. Having an updated last will and testament will ensure that assets and other property will be divided after their death according to their wishes. Power of attorney documents are also important if the older adult should reach a point where they are no longer able to make their own health care or legal decisions.
- Completion of these documents should help to minimize the stress associated with an emergency and maximize the quality of the care the older adult receives.

Task Question: Have you encouraged your parent to consult with an elder law attorney to be sure legal documents represent their wishes?

Learn More: Understanding Legal Documents

- A will, power of attorney, and/or trust agreements should be executed while the older adult is competent; otherwise, a court action is required to transfer the responsibility for management of the financial affairs to another person.

- Because the documents are often complex, it is recommended that older adults complete them while they are healthy and able to discuss their preferences with children, family members, and other possible decision-makers.

- After documents are completed, they should be shared with family members, physicians, and clergy to be sure they are entered into the medical record in case the older adult is hospitalized. It is also important to keep these documents secured in a fireproof safe and/or a secure electronic vault.

Wills

- A will is a legal document that incorporates a financial inventory and states how property and assets should be distributed upon death.

- If the older adult does not have a will, you should encourage them to consult an attorney. A will does not override beneficiary designations stated in certain documents (insurance policies, bank accounts, and annuities), so it is usually better to specifically name beneficiaries for these types of accounts and policies instead of simply stating that the proceeds be made payable to the older adult's estate.

- A well-executed will reduces the likelihood of family conflicts over funeral and burial decisions, as well as conflicts over the distribution of material goods. A periodic review of an existing will is necessary when there are tax law changes, if there has been an out-of-state move, a purchase of out-of-state property, marriage, divorce, birth, education needs, health needs, and/or charity involvement.

Trusts

- A trust is a legal agreement that allows a third party the right to hold and direct benefits on behalf of a beneficiary. Trust agreements are particularly useful to insure uninterrupted property management, particularly if property is owned in multiple states.
- A person who creates the trust is the grantor, the person who manages the trust is the trustee, and the person who benefits from the trust is the beneficiary. In a revocable trust, the older adult may serve as the grantor, trustee, and the beneficiary. An alternate trustee can take over when the older adult can no longer manage the property.
- Upon death, generally without probate, the property can be distributed to one or more designated beneficiaries. Once the trust is established, property must be conveyed to the trust by signing and recording deeds for real estate. For bank accounts and other titled property, including insurance policies and vehicles, the assets must be transferred and retitled in the name of the trustee.

Power of Attorney

- A power of attorney is a legal document that gives a chosen person legal authority to act on another person's behalf. Setting this up is a fairly simple process and is important to do while the older adult is physically and mentally healthy to ensure their wishes are followed.
- It should be noted that if the older adult has signed a power of attorney and later becomes incompetent by way of dementia, Alzheimer's, illness, or accident, the power of attorney is automatically terminated. To avoid this situation, we recommend a durable power of attorney that will remain in effect regardless of any potential incapacity.
- A springing power of attorney makes the authority effective on a certain date in the future, or upon the occurrence of a particular event such as disability or incapacity. This is a good option if the older adult isn't ready to give over their rights today but wants to be prepared for the future.

Power of Attorney Options

- It is important to note that there are different types of these documents, and having both will ensure the older adult is fully covered in the event they become unable to make decisions on their own.
- A health care power of attorney is needed to develop advance directives for care and will appoint someone to make health care decisions on their behalf.
- A legal power of attorney is needed to act on the older adult's behalf on legal and financial manners like paying bills and accessing assets.

Advance Directives for Health Care

- Living will: A living will is a legal document that tells doctors how you want to be treated if you cannot make your own decisions about emergency treatment. In a living will, you can say which common medical treatments or care you would want, which ones you would want to avoid, and under which conditions each of your choices applies.
- Durable power of attorney for health care: A durable power of attorney for health care is a legal document that names your health care proxy, a person who can make health care decisions for you if you are unable to communicate these yourself. Your proxy, also known as a representative, surrogate, or agent, should be familiar with your values and wishes. A proxy can be chosen in addition to or instead of a living will. Having a health care proxy helps you plan for situations that cannot be foreseen, such as a serious car accident or stroke. Think of your advance directives as living documents that you review at least once each year and update if a major life event occurs such as retirement, moving out of state, or a significant change in your health.

Resources

- National Academy of Elder Law Attorneys, on finding an elder law attorney (https://www.naela.org/findlawyer)
- Family Caregiver Alliance, on finding a lawyer for estate planning; also includes information on important legal documents for seniors

(https://www.caregiver.org/resource/finding-attorney-help-estate-planning/?via=caregiver-resources,all-resources)
- National Institute on Aging, on planning an advance directive for health care (https://www.nia.nih.gov/health/advance-care-planning-advance-directives-health-care)
- Alabama Public Health, on an advance directive for use in Alabama—be sure to check the requirements for your own state (https://www.alabamapublichealth.gov/cancer/assets/advdirective.pdf)
- Alabama Department of Senior Services, on finding legal assistance for Alabama seniors (https://alabamaageline.gov/legal-assistance/)

Other Legal-Financial Domain Topics

- Budget plan
- Exploring benefits
- Long-term care plan
- Property review
- Family heirlooms
- Care of dependents
- Fraud prevention
- Organizational elements

Family-Social Tasks

As people age, they often need help from family members due to chronic health conditions, mobility limitations, and sensory changes. Caregiving is a family affair, and social support from family and friends is crucial in successfully navigating these challenges. As a middle-aged child, it's important to plan carefully with aging parents, spouses, siblings, and other members of their social convoy to ensure adequate support.

Task Name: Family Meeting
Task Overview

- Organizing a family meeting to discuss the care of the older adult is a vital step in preparedness for their future care. It is important to consider a family approach, including blended family members, when planning for the older adult's future care.
- This is a time to discuss how everyone can work together in preserving the older adult's independence and dignity in the face of possible limitations. It is also a time to learn more about the older adult's current physical health, health insurance, resources available for his/her care, and the plans the older adult has made for advance directives.
- Some families may find it useful to ask a geriatric care manager or other nonfamily member (clergy member, close family friend) to facilitate the discussion.

Task Question: Have you convened a family meeting to develop an initial plan about how each person can be involved in caring for the older adult?

Learn More: Tips on Holding a Successful Family Meeting

- Decide who will be responsible for specific tasks. You can even name a primary caregiver who will be responsible for orchestrating things in the event of an emergency.
- Discuss strengths and weaknesses when delegating caregiving responsibilities and tasks. Finding out what each person is good at can be very helpful in planning for the future. Some people are good at managing finances, while others would be better suited to dealing with medical tasks.
- Consider everyone's limits and boundaries, and be realistic about how much you can and are willing to do. It is important to understand the responsibility of taking on caregiving duties.
- If you or other family members live in a different area than the older adult, you'll want to discuss the ways you can help support them. There are things that you don't need to be present for like giving emotional support, arranging for professional caregivers, researching options for care, or providing financial support or managing finances.

Resources

- Family Caregiver Alliance, on holding a family meeting (https://www.caregiver.org/resource/holding-family-meeting/)
- National Institute on Aging, on how to share caregiving responsibilities with family members (https://www.nia.nih.gov/health/caregiving/sharing-caregiving-responsibilities)
- Family Caregiver Alliance, on caregiving with your siblings (https://www.caregiver.org/resource/caregiving-with-your-siblings/?via=caregiver-resources,all-resources)
- National Institute on Aging, on long-distance caregiving (https://www.nia.nih.gov/health/long-distance-caregiving/what-long-distance-caregiving)
- Geriatric Fast Facts, on tips for leading difficult family meetings (https://www.geriatricfastfacts.com/fast-facts/tips-leading-difficult-family-meetings)

Other Family-Social Domain Topics

- Meetings
- Companion animals
- Planning
- Using technology
- Home safety
- Personal caregiving
- Grandparenting
- Home maintenance
- Widowhood support

Spiritual-Emotional Tasks

To keep older adults healthy, it is important to include spirituality and emotions in health promotion models. Spirituality and religion are important for many older adults and can help them cope with life events. Religion can also help people deal with mental health and substance abuse issues. Being involved in religion can provide social support and offer a sense of hope and meaning in life. Children of older adults can help their parents by completing tasks that improve their spiritual and emotional well-being.

Task Name: Capturing Your Older Adult's Story
Task Overview

- Reminiscence and life review approaches have been developed specifically for older adults and their families to help them find meaning through describing and discussing memories of their life experiences. This can help in achieving a sense of meaning to one's life by preparing a legacy for after the older adult has passed.
- Sharing and documenting this information with friends and family members, especially younger ones such as grandchildren, can help to keep the older adult's memories alive for years to come. This can be done through a written account of stories or audio/video recordings of the older adult recounting their life experiences.

Task Question: Have you captured the older adult's story where s/he talks about various life experiences, including military service, and shares advice for the future with children, grandchildren, and other members of the family?

Learn More: Suggestions and Ideas for Documenting

Create a List of Questions

- What are some things you wish you had been able to ask older family members before they passed? What are things you would want others to know about you when you're gone? Asking yourself these questions can help to develop a list of talking points to discuss with the older adult.
- This can also be helpful if the older adult is unsure what to talk about or is hesitant/shy to discuss their life experiences.

Family Values

- The transmission of family values can be accomplished by encouraging older adults to document what is really important in their lives (intergenerational transfers of wisdom and faith).

Life Stories, Whether They Are Everyday Experiences or Special Events

- Everyone has a story to tell. Getting to know an older adult through reminiscing can help family members discover many positive qualities they had never realized or appreciated.

Future Messages and Advice for Younger Family Members

- Consider recording future messages and advice from the older adult to younger members (or yet-to-be-born members) of the family around significant events that have not happened yet. They can also record messages to share with grandchildren on future special occasions.
- Topics can include religious events, high school and college graduations, engagement and marriage, birth of great-grandchildren, selecting a career, gaining a driving license, and more. They can also include tougher, difficult subjects like drinking, drugs, and depression.

Resources

- Smithsonian Institution Archives, on how to do oral history (https://siarchives.si.edu/history/how-do-oral-history)
- Library of Congress, on oral histories (https://loc.gov/folklife/family-folklife/oralhistory.html)
- Senior Advisor, on a guide for interviewing elders (https://www.senioradvisor.com/blog/2014/09/the-power-of-sharing-life-stories-a-step-by-step-guide-and-resources-for-interviewing-our-elders/)
- National Museum of African American History and Culture, on capturing the oral history of your family (https://nmaahc.si.edu/explore/stories/capturing-your-familys-oral-history)

Other Spiritual-Social Domain Topics

- Funeral wishes and plans
- End of life care
- Making peace/blessing children, grands, and great-grands
- Spiritual beliefs, needs, and strengths
- Local and internet faith-based programs targeting older people and their caregivers
- Discover and affirm late-life purpose
- Church and family network/convoy

Chapter 14

The Gift of Blessing the Next Generation

FOR MANY OF US, when we think of blessing in the Christian realm, the story of Jacob and Esau comes to mind: twin brothers who fought over the birthright and blessing from their father. While we might relegate this idea to Old Testament Scripture, the concept is still very current in our lives today. Over the years I (Jim) have had students in my office, sharing their aches and yearnings to feel accepted and loved by their parents or siblings. The relationship that we had with our parents can affect future relationships with others and the way that we see ourselves. God has created us for intimacy. The very nature of how God has created us contributes to this. A baby nursing at the mother's breast is the exact distance that the child can see the mother's face in focus. That intimate relationship of mother and child is enhanced by eye-to-eye contact. If the mother does not look on the child, the child suffers from the lack of intimacy and acceptance. That suffering can carry on into other relationships as the child grows and can be a destructive element. So too the child will look for acceptance and love from the father figure. This may be a birth father but can also be found in grandparents or mature males who take on this role.

Accepting our children and passing on a blessing to them is of utmost importance and can be such a gift. We may not have been able to provide the kind of blessing that they are looking for, but we have tried to see and acknowledge their gifts and abilities, and to celebrate them as the Lord has made them to be. Part of passing on a blessing is to pray for them and with them. In prayer we all humble ourselves before the Living God and recognize our need to be loved and accepted first by him. It is in his grace that we are able to see ourselves as free and deeply loved. As humans, though, we also need words of affirmation and touch. It has always been my joy to hug my own children, but also hug (in an appropriate manner) those who are brokenhearted—to meet their needs emotionally but also to give a tangible act of acceptance.

A couple of years ago I (Jim) had a vision that, in my ninety-ninth year, the Lord was calling me home. My children gathered about my bed, and we held hands, being physically connected. I prayed for each of them by name, seeing their unique personhood and abilities. This was my way of passing on a blessing to each of them. I also wrote a letter to each of my grandchildren that is to be given to them at my passing. In these letters I have again tried to see each child as they are, with their strengths and gifts, and lifted them up to the Lord for him to bless them mightily. As a mere man I will not do this perfectly, and the recipients may not be able to receive them in the vein meant, but I have tried to love and affirm them as I can. I pray that the Spirit will interpret as promised and will pass on what is in my heart, putting it into words that they can see and accept.

In your final years don't wait or lose the opportunity to bless your children, grandchildren, and even great-grandchildren. There may have been a lot of painful history, but now is the time to seek to make those amends. God is abounding in grace and strength, and he is just waiting to pour it out for us. For further information on the topic of intergenerational blessing, we recommend Dr. John Trent's book, *The Blessing*.[1]

---

1. Trent et al., *Blessing*.

Epilogue[1]

Jim Houston's Farewell Letter Written on the Eve of His Hundredth Birthday

Blessed is the man
who walks not in the counsel of the wicked,
nor stands in the way of sinners,
nor sits in the seat of scoffers;
but his delight is in the law of the Lord,
and on his law he meditates day and night.
He is like a tree
planted by streams of water,
that yields its fruit in its season,
and its leaf does not wither.
In all that he does, he prospers.
The wicked are not so,
but are like chaff which the wind drives away.
Therefore the wicked will not stand in the judgment,
nor sinners in the congregation of the righteous;
for the Lord knows the way of the righteous,
but the way of the wicked will perish.
(Ps 1 RSV)

---

1. *Letters from a Hospital Bed* is a series of reflections by Jim Houston, now entering his hundredth year, in which Jim seeks to capture and reflect new insights of his ever-discoverable God, revealed through his own hospitalization, for the encouragement of all caregivers. See https://www.jimhouston.org/blog and scroll down to find individual letters. This letter was written by Jim in collaboration with his son, Chris Houston.

Dear Friends:

In just a few days from now, on November 21st, I will celebrate my 100th birthday. My mother, to whom I was born when she was forty years of age, had been told at the age of eighteen that she had but a few years to live. So much for prognostications about life expectancy! It seems her genes and those of my father were tougher than expected. But this milestone causes me to ask more than a few times, "Why did God spare me to now, to live for over a century instead of my 'allotment' of 'three score years and ten'? And what could I say to my friends at a time like this?"

I have outlived *all* my peers and colleagues and nearly *all* my friends from my own generation—though clearly not any of you who are still reading my letters! Just over a year ago, I entered this hospital, also a hospice, where dear Rita had died and where I hoped to soon follow her. So certain and so eager was I to return to the Lord that I gave my children instructions concerning my funeral arrangements, including the substitution of a traditional photograph with the version of Ps 1 that I have shared with you before and which is reproduced above.

The psalmist David uses this psalm as the entry point into the transparency of his heart before God, which unfolds through the poetry that follows. The image you see with this letter hangs before my table as I write, with the bed in which I will likely breathe my last on one side and a window out to the adjacent park filled with vibrant life on the other. Here I sit before the psalm, slung between my own eternal rest and the continuity of life outside my window. The literary center of the psalm before me, its focus, its heart, is the simple word *fruit*. Fruit that is borne by the well-rooted tree through the choices of one that follows the way of the righteous. A third of the poems that follow in the psalms are laments.

Many psalms contain language that seems wholly inappropriate, even rude, unless they are being spoken, in deep distress and honesty, to a loving and personal God who really wants to hear what we say. This book, this word, is where I choose to focus my attention as I give thanks for the grace of one hundred years, such that it may one day be said that my life was fruitful. Not until we arrive at the New Testament text do we really understand the nature of the fruitful life promised for the well-rooted tree. The apostle Paul, writing his letter to the Galatians, describes what these fruits are; they are: "love, joy, peace, forbearance, kindness, goodness, faithfulness, and self-control." So that when we are in the presence of others, our "presence" can become "a therapeutic presence" for others.

EPILOGUE

The early fathers saw the fruits as being from the healing of our souls, that Jesus Christ has become our Eternal Physician, and through his healing of us, we become bearers of the fruit of his Spirit. None of us yet are fully "healed," but the journey to "soul health" is now in progress, until in the eternal presence of his glory, we shall be like him, fully healed, fully fruitful. Then we shall be restored to be God's delight, like his Beloved Son, who at his baptism was as acclaimed as being well pleasing to his Father. Importantly, these fruits listed by the apostle, which we should produce, are not us, but from us.

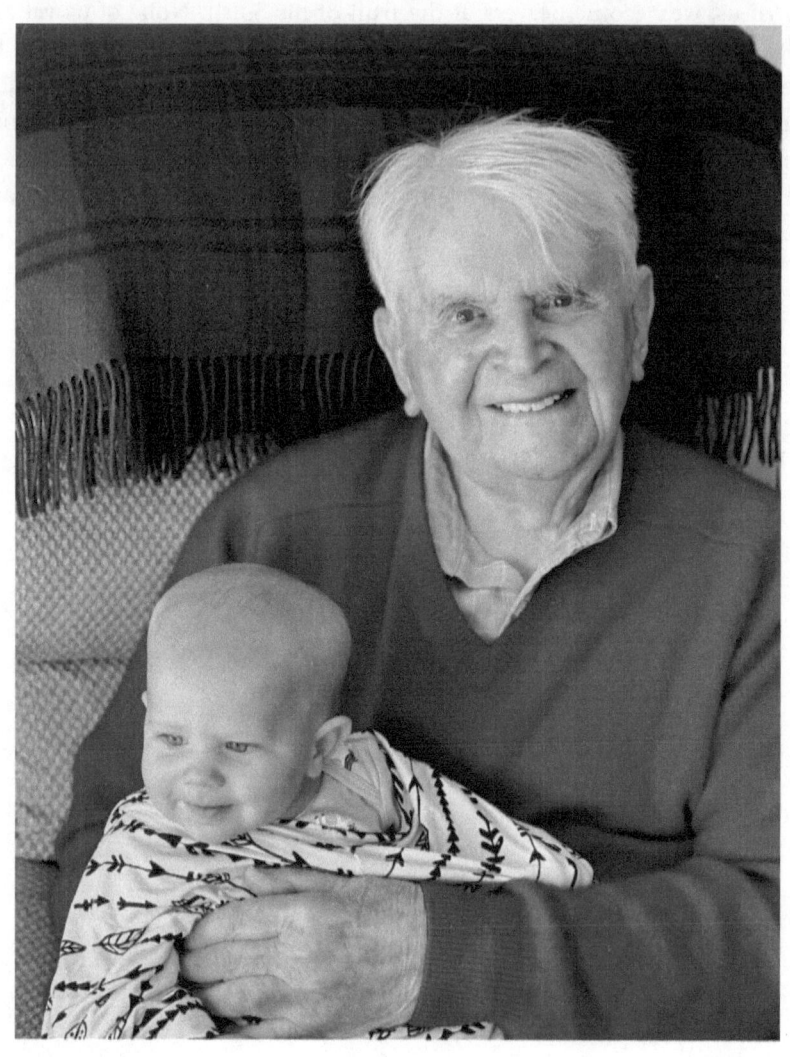

Jim with his youngest great-grandchild, Heidi.

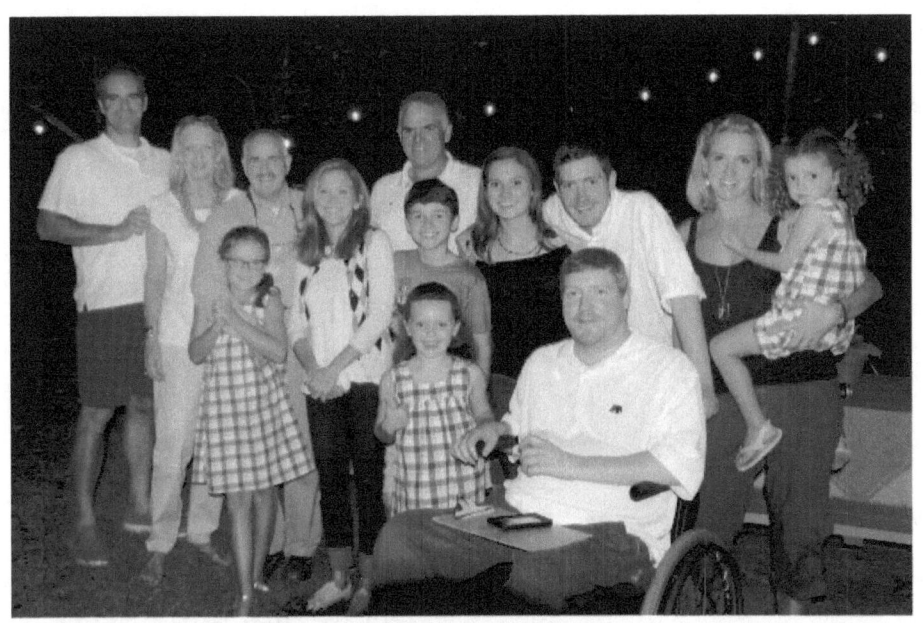

The Parker family on Mike's seventy-fifth birthday.

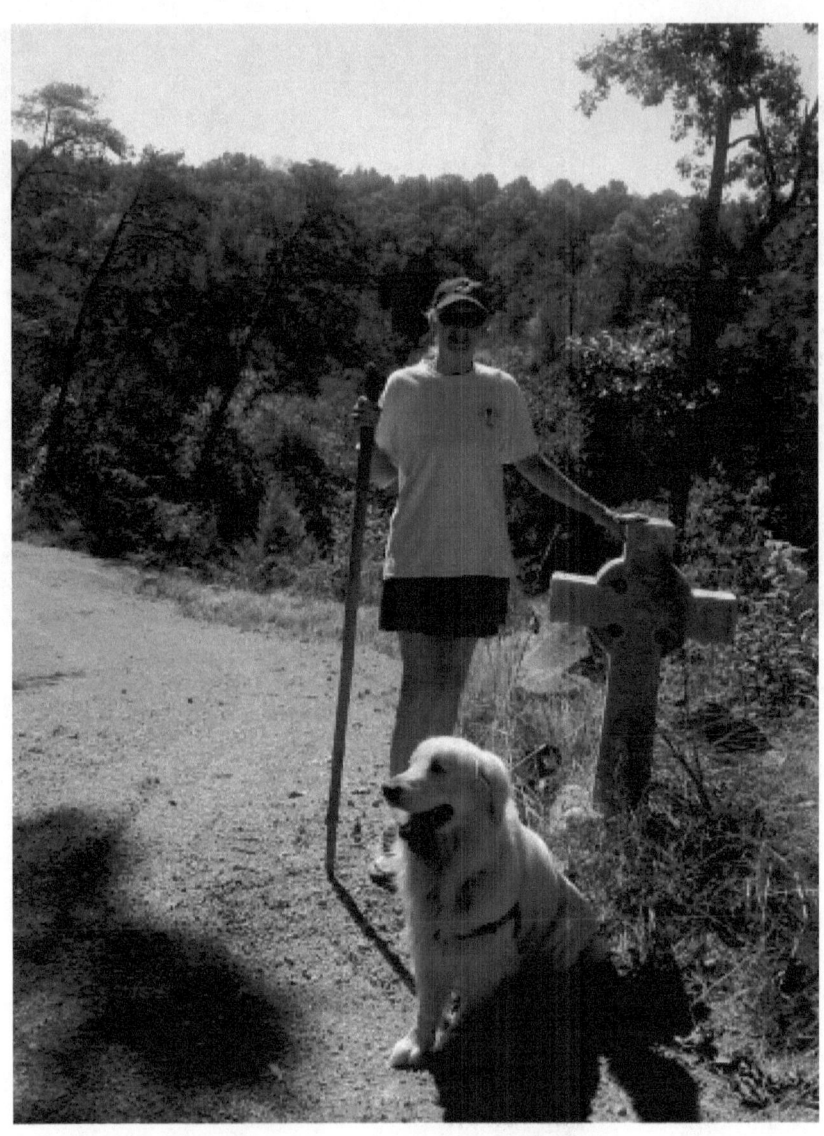

Mike's wife, Lane, with their dog Champ.

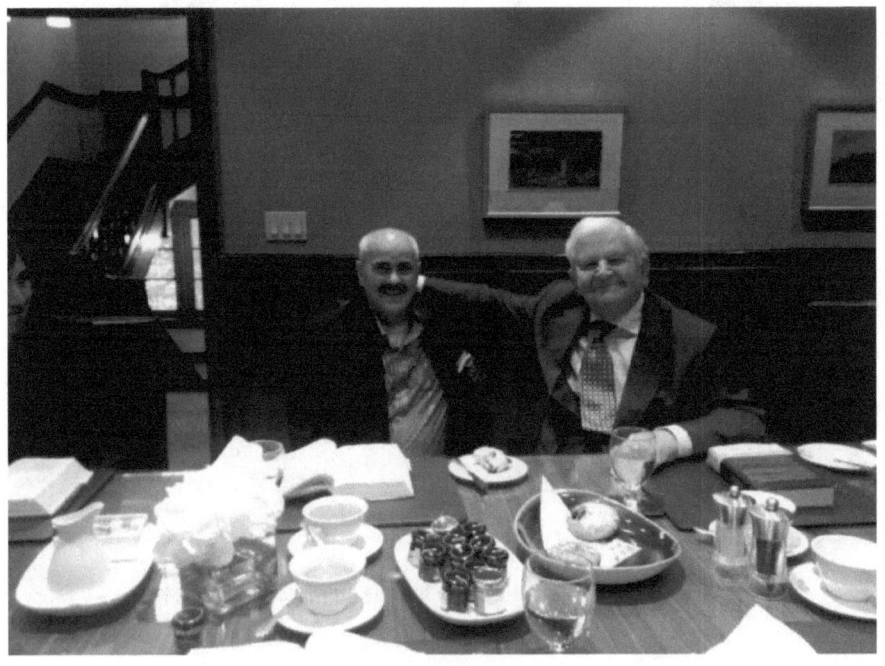

Jim and Mike together at dinner in Vancouver in 2018.

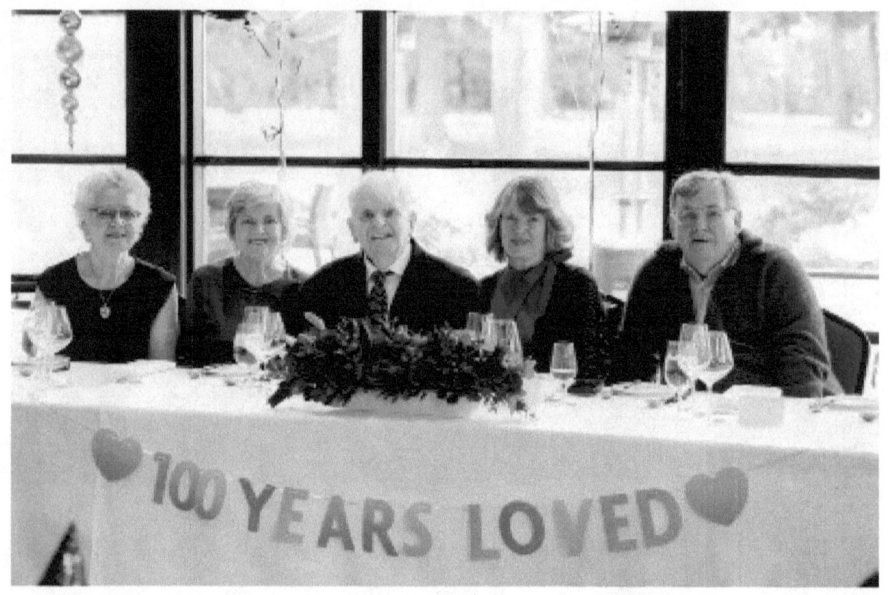

Jim with his adult children on his one hundredth birthday.

Appendices
Faith-Based Programs

Appendix A
Introduction

INTRODUCTION: CHURCH PROGRAMS FOR SENIORS AND THOSE WHO CARE FOR THEM

In the appendix that follows, we discuss a range of age-friendly, biblically informed, programs that help congregations and individuals respond to the aging imperative faced by the church, our nation, and most of the world. Since our first book (*A Vision for the Aging Church: Renewing Ministry for and by Seniors*), we have received over a thousand email messages, multiple requests to speak at Christian and professional conferences, hundreds of phone calls, and over twenty site visits from pastors and business leaders. We have worked with military chaplains, conducted elder care research with congregations, and completed a clinical trial with a parent care readiness program at the U.S. Air War College and a longitudinal survey of senior-ranking military officers' (assigned to the U.S. Army War College) distant caregiving experiences. We have been encouraged to see signs of great progress by the church and in seminaries, where our first book is being used to introduce the topic of aging.

On a strategic level, the James Houston Center is working with military chaplains regarding the adoption of a new mission, in keeping with the fifth commandment of preparing active-duty service members for parent/elder care. Research has shown that male and female careerists are particularly vulnerable to severe stress associated with long-distance parent care.[1] The Houston Center has also supported faith-based systems that have assisted vulnerable elderly persons following disasters (e.g., the Russian invasion of Ukraine, recent tornadoes in the south, COVID pandemic) with

---

1. Parker et al., "'Out of Sight.'"

an age-friendly triage system developed by a Baylor University team following Hurricane Katrina. Older and disabled people are highly vulnerable to disasters that require significant change and adjustment.

Our reason for including descriptions of promising ministries is to provide local communities and congregations with programs that meet genuine needs now, and to promote and expand these viable ministries. By "thinking globally and acting locally," using the internet and technologies like Zoom, we hope that some congregations, communities, and individuals will use the information included here to start new needed programs for elders.

From a dementia respite program for fatigued family caregivers to a new program that honors aging veterans, we have included a variety of new and well-established programs for your consideration. In some cases, you can simply link up with an existing program, like GrandsMatter, that encourages and supports Christian grandparents and great-grandparents. Or perhaps you want to build on an existing program that helps adult children prepare for the care of their aging parents. Included are projects by senior ministry associations that describe faith and successful aging conferences, an age-friendly resource development project, and an elder care study at two congregations. We encourage you to review carefully each of the programs included here and to take note of the training and experience of those who manage these programs. Using modern technologies and our relationships with these new leaders, we aim to help you, the church, and other faith-based organizations to "link up" with these committed Christian leaders and ministries and to start new needed programs.

Our aging is something that all of us share but many deny, yet God appears to be allowing us to live longer—and we believe in our innermost being—for an eternal purpose. In reviewing the information in these appendices, we hope you will see how the church can lead the way in building age-friendly programs that demonstrate the love of Christ, help promote existing programs, fill gaps in service, and identify new resources. As Daphne Johnston would say about her prestigious, award-winning dementia respite program for family caregivers, her teams of volunteers take the love of Christ to touch the lives of families at a point of great need. Through other programs, like the congregational veterans program designed by Colonel Martin's distinguished teams of experts, veterans can be honored and find healing in a supportive group atmosphere that uses "life review" and the creative arts to capture their stories.

Family caregivers are often isolated; elders are depressed and alone; professionals hold conferences for their respective professions, all the while vast numbers of our congregations and neighbors have no idea how to age successfully or to provide care to an elderly loved one suffering from one of the dreaded dementias. Professionals in the growing field of aging call it *translational research* . . . sharing what we know with those who need this lifesaving, life-enhancing information. Based upon correspondence from hundreds of readers of our earlier book, we think churches with improved sensitivity to the needs of older people and those who care for them can apply research that can help older people to age successfully when supported by knowledgeable professionals like those who have contributed to this appendix. We have tried to focus specifically on important, often neglected topics and to provide a hands-on informational guide about how to develop/implement much-needed programs successfully. Considerable progress has been made since our last book was published, and we remain committed to sharing the good news about Christ and effective age-friendly ministries. Thinking globally, yet acting locally, can help our churches become more age friendly. Our view is that older persons are a gift, not a burden, to the church. We posit that longer life represents an opportunity for Christian older persons and those who care for them to make a difference through Holy Spirit-inspired ministries.

Appendix B
Faith-Based Initiatives in Support of America's Veterans

THIS REPORT IS INTENDED to promote the development of faith-based programs for veterans in churches, synagogues, mosques, and other religious centers in the United States. The goal is to encourage members of faith communities to recognize, honor, and support America's veterans, whose military service and sacrifice often go unrecognized, and whose well-being would likely benefit from a faith connection. The intent is to leverage the power of faith communities to offer recognition and various forms of social-emotional connection and support to aging veterans and their caregivers.

According to a 2021 report of the Pew Research Center, there are approximately 19 million US veterans. Fewer than 240,000 of these veterans served in World War II, and about 933,000 served during the Korean conflict.[2] These represent America's oldest veterans. Approximately 5.9 million veterans served during the Vietnam era, and most are now in their seventies. Thirty-six percent of veterans are between fifty and sixty-nine years of age, and 37 percent are age seventy or older. About one in ten veterans are women. Over the next few decades, the percentage of women veterans is expected to increase slightly. Today, 74 percent of veterans are non-Hispanic White; 8 percent are Hispanic; and 13 percent are Black. The percentage of Hispanic veterans is likely to double in the next few decades, the percent of Black veterans will increase slightly, while the number of non-Hispanic

---

2. Schaeffer, "Changing Face."

White veterans will decline during this period to around 64 percent of all veterans.

Not all veterans served in combat. Some never deployed to a war zone, and those who served in a war zone may not have seen combat. Still, many who served in a war zone, especially in the recent wars in Afghanistan and Iraq, are likely to have found very little distinction between combat and non-combat experiences. The violence and trauma of war may have reached a veteran even if he or she was not officially engaged in combat. Many veterans were exposed to trauma through military operations other than war (MOOTW), including military disaster responses. Also, many veterans of the National Guard and the other reserve components were exposed to combat, as well as to MOOTW service. Veterans who were never deployed to a war zone may have experienced challenging physical and/or psychological conditions associated with their military service life.

All veterans may experience adverse psychosocial outcomes like substance use disorders, housing instability, and/or food insecurity as they age. Illness, accidents, and interpersonal violence, among other stress and trauma exposures, may be part of a veteran's earlier military experience, and the emotional baggage of military service often weighs heavily in a veteran's civilian rucksack.

Many aging veterans depend on family or other caregivers, and programs to serve veterans need to recognize the influence of caregivers on the veteran's life and well-being. The nature and quality of caregiving can influence health and psychosocial outcomes like loneliness, social isolation, and substance use disorders and can have a profound impact on the veteran's personal narrative. Thus, faith-based interventions need to include ways to connect with and support the veteran's caregiver as well.

Faith-based communities have a wonderful opportunity to honor and support our veterans and their caregivers. Congregations can also promote intergenerational dialogue and offer older veterans an opportunity to share their important life stories with younger generations in a setting of care and compassion.

Churches, synagogues, mosques, and other religious centers may initiate or further develop veteran outreach initiatives specifically targeted at older veterans, both in their congregations and in their communities. Younger veterans (and veterans' family members) in the congregation may lead these efforts. Communities of faith have the opportunity to recognize veterans on various holidays and support worthy veteran organizations in the local community. Discussion groups, particularly those focused on life review, would offer older veterans an opportunity to share stories of their military service as well as their post-service life experiences with younger generations. These are but a few of many possibilities that faith-based communities may develop as part of a ministry directed at our nation's veterans.

References

1. Swords to Plowshares, "Quick Facts."
2. Spiro et al., "Long-Term Outcomes."
3. Fogle et al., "National Health and Resilience."

Resources

Veterans Socials (https://www.mentalhealth.va.gov/socials/index.asp)

Veteran Resources (https://www.mentalhealth.va.gov/older-veterans/resources.asp)

Appendix C
The Eric Liddell Community of Today

CARE. COMPASSION. COMMUNITY.

Our vision is to live in a community where no one feels lonely or isolated, and we're on a mission to bring people together in their local community to improve health and well-being and have a positive impact on their lives.

Our three-core program—support for people living with dementia, support for unpaid carers, and running a thriving community hub—have always been the heartbeat of our mission. The Eric Liddell Community was founded in memory of the 1924 Olympic four-hundred meter gold medalist, Scottish international rugby player, and committed missionary Eric Liddell, as the need for care, compassion, and community was made known in Edinburgh.

Our Values

At the Eric Liddell Community we are:

- Compassionate: We care for each other and our community.
- Respectful: We treat everyone with dignity.
- Inclusive: We ensure fair treatment and opportunity for all.
- People Centered: We keep our community at the heart of everything we do.
- Sustainable: We look after our people and our planet.
- Led by Integrity: We keep our promises.

Strategic Priorities

- Grow our service for people living with dementia
- Extend our program for unpaid caregivers
- Develop a community hub that supports the needs of our local community
- Develop and celebrate the legacy of Eric Liddell

Our Services

Support for people living with dementia. We run a varied program of support for people living with dementia, including our flagship day care service, to help ensure older people can fulfill their potential with dignity and equality and in a healthy environment. Our support offers people living with dementia, whatever their stage of diagnosis, and their families the chance for vital respite. It strives to enable people living with dementia to stay in their homes for longer by improving the quality of their lives through excellent care and support.

Support for unpaid caregivers. Our varied program of support for unpaid caregivers includes free health and well-being classes, lunch breaks, music therapy, and befriending across Edinburgh. The program provides vital opportunities for caregivers to take a short break from their caring role as well as opportunities for caregivers and the person they care for to partake jointly in activities that help revive and sustain their relationship.

Appendix D
A Short History of the Eric Liddell Centre/Community

ORIGINS

At the heart of the capital of the most beautiful country in the world towers a castle that has witnessed the unfolding of history through the rule of kings and queens, changes brought about by the Reformation, the Enlightenment, and the rumbling Old Town enhanced by the wide boulevards of the New Town. The vistas that it beholds include seats of learning, galleries, museums, monuments, finance houses, theaters, government buildings, law courts, and many vast and beautiful parklands. Edinburgh lays claim to celebrated authors, poets, politicians, theologians, sportsmen and women, and, of course, Nobel Prize winners. Festivals and celebrations draw folks from all over the globe, people who know that what they experience there will be special to them forever.

To the southwest of the castle, there is a crossroads where Bruntsfield, Chamberlain Road, Morningside Road, and Colinton Road all meet. On each corner of this crossroads stands a church, giving the crossroads the forever name of Holy Corner. The churches, certainly at the commencement of this story, were from very different theological backgrounds: North Morningside Parish Church; Morningside Baptist Church; Christchurch Morningside; and the Congregational Church, Morningside. Now whether by eternal design, the fury of mother nature, carelessness, or bad plumbing, I do not know, but three of the four would suffer catastrophes caused by flood, wind, and fire, forcing the congregations to use the only remaining disaster-free church for their worship and service.

Over the months, as inspections, tenders, and repairs took place, the congregations found common purpose through joint worship, prayer, Bible study, and, importantly, service. It was their service to the wider community that would draw them closer still as they realized that they shared the same concerns and care for the unemployed, hurting, and most vulnerable elderly people around them. They had been responding, of course, but decided that these Christian acts of love could be better achieved if they worked together. So they did.

The members of North Morningside Parish Church and the Congregational Church decided that rather than simply sharing concern and care for others, they would like to follow God's guidance into a much fuller union of the congregations. This would come to pass under the aegis of an act of Parliament, leaving a redundant building. Wise counsel was sought, and it was agreed that the North Morningside Parish Church would be sold. The Holy Corner Christians, envisioning the possibilities that lay ahead, created a charitable organization that was conditional on one third of each of the members of the three congregations pledging to support it. This objective was met as members entered into a covenant to finance, manage, and serve in the newly formed charity. The redundant premises were purchased using a short-term loan from the recently formed Morningside United Church. The Holy Corner Churches Centre now had premises that provided a base for their increasing workload in the community. Wisely, the churches retained the evangelical outreach for the locality and supported a charitable constitution with clearly stated social and community objectives.

When pews, organ, pulpit, and choir stalls were removed and "ticky-tacky" boxes created walls for semi-permanent offices, service to the community expanded from lunch clubs and a friendship group to include Christian healing, pastoral care and counseling, educational activities, an executive job club, and an innovative one-on-one day care service for people with a diagnosis of dementia on one day each week. During this decade of expansion, amid the spectrum of light coming from the saints surrounding them, leaders organized an architectural competition that would result in a design to match their vision for the future of the building itself.

Of course, it wasn't all smooth sailing. There were fallouts, squabbles, power struggles, celebrations, and, of necessity, the occasional service of reconciliation and forgiveness as well as thanksgiving for progress made. The architectural competition was won by Nicholas Groves-Raines, and coterminous with a change of name to the Eric Liddell Centre, a fundraising appeal commenced in the early 1990s. Eric Henry Liddell, world-famous athlete, rugby player, and missionary, recently commemorated in the award-winning film *Chariots of Fire*, had worshiped and taught Bible class in the Congregational Church while studying at the University of Edinburgh. In fact, his service of dedication to missionary work took place there just prior to his leaving for China, and some members of the center could remember attending it. While there are conflicting stories about where the idea to rename the center came from, it was clear that this community had an international hero and exemplar whom they wanted to honor and emulate.

BUILDING FOR THE COMMUNITY

It is said that the best-laid schemes "gang aft aglay," and so it was that having completed phase 1 of work to complete a center on five floors within the cocoon of the historic building, work had to be brought to a halt. Inflation in the cost of building materials, relocation of the boiler house to the exterior of the building, and finding the hollowed-out remains of an ancient cesspit that required infilling with ton upon ton of unbudgeted and costly concrete caused a deficit of over £100,000 in the scheme. The scheme had to be put on hold until additional funding could be found. Potential funders refused to provide further support until they could see some form of positive outcome related to the investments they had already made. Some of the members and trustees believed that having gotten the basic structure in place and having completed the ground floor, it was unlikely they would see completion in their lifetimes. The whole project seemed doomed.

It was into this situation that the three churches, in addition to the regular annual support that they provided, promised to give additional financial support over two years to create a new post. This sacrificial investment in the center and the community's future would prove pivotal. A previous short-term post had provided some research finds, which, unfortunately, had not been written up. This work had been commissioned to verify that the advice received from members about the way forward was correct and to ensure that there could be no accusation of irrelevant care being parachuted into the community.

Despite the failure to complete, there was a buzz in the community about the building's being named after a local hero and a curiosity about what it would be like and what it would do when completed. Detailed relationship building with key community leaders and opinion makers began, and out of many meaningful discussions over lunch or coffee, a community desire to help grew. This took the form of the 3Ms Research Project (Marchmont, Merchiston, and Morningside wards), which was formed with a membership of three local City of Edinburgh councillors; the local member of parliament; representatives from the three community councils; local charity managers; and representatives from churches, health, social work, and education.

The research area in which the Eric Liddell Centre sat was to be one in seven of twenty-one thousand homes in the three wards. A professional researcher was employed, and work began on designing, printing, and disseminating via the postal service a social needs survey to be completed and written up by the end of 1996. If successful, the research would provide valuable information that would be crucial to the ongoing development of services within the wider community. The anticipated return rate was 10 to 12 percent.

The return rate for the survey was overwhelming at 28 percent. Volunteers were recruited to assist the researcher. They were managed by a worker seconded from the Community Education Department. The findings confirmed that the anticipated growth trajectory for specialist day care provision for people with a diagnosis of dementia would be greater than expected and that the pilot project that had provided short respite breaks for caregivers must be expanded. Other findings related to a lack of youth provision in the area, and to the loneliness and isolation of retired women living on their own with lower pensions than their male counterparts. The study also found that there was no need to develop additional services for people with mental health problems.

The findings of the social needs survey were the impetus that the center needed. The survey not only provided proof of need, but became the dynamic force integral to all funding applications to complete the building, empowered by the necessity for a specialist day care unit at the heart of the community. Plans for the future included a floor to provide day care services. Offices would provide a base from which an innovative citywide service for caregivers would be run.

SPECIALIST DAY CARE FOR PEOPLE WITH A DIAGNOSIS OF DEMENTIA

Key to the success of any project is the personnel. The Eric Liddell Centre's day care service has always been blessed with highly professional volunteers and staff. The early days of the service, which had developed from one to two days as the need arose, utilized trained volunteers to work on an individual basis with each client when activities necessitated it. This exemplary model of care was designed and implemented by an excellent mental health nurse who was employed to lead the project. Such was the quality of the service that it was included as an exemplar of good practice in a Europe-wide study of different care models.

While the newly completed facility became the base for the day care services for eight persons each Tuesday and Thursday, the center also developed an outreach service in the Tollcross area. This was provided on Mondays and Wednesdays in the common room of a housing association but used professionally trained staff.

The introduction of the Care Inspectorate meant considerable change to meet the stringent quality standards set by the inspectorate. Unfortunately, it wasn't possible to continue using the common room, so an agreement was made that this outreach provision would move into the day care unit at the center. This move necessitated an integration and streamlining of the two, which melded happily under the staffing model. These important changes took place with the support of a specialist day care committee to which the center board had delegated responsibility for staffing and development.

Development continued as the need for the service grew. Eventually services were added on Fridays. Then numbers each day grew to twelve, and with Care Inspectorate permission, to fourteen places. A Snoezelen Room was funded by one of the three churches, and a reminiscence room was created to trigger memories and support activities.

The day care experience was a joy to participate in. Clients arrived by the transport provided and on arrival sat down to breakfast and the companionship of other clients, staff, and volunteers. Activities such as quizzes, games, dance, exercise, and singing were the basis for fun and conversation, with special events seen as essential ingredients on the calendar. For those who desired, there was the opportunity, twice monthly, to attend worship that had been carefully designed to take maximum support to the clients. The chaplain was included in all major events and was deeply appreciated, not only by the clients, but also by their caregivers and other family members.

CA(I)RE—PUTTING THE *I* INTO CARE

This project began when I attended a conference where I heard caregivers speak about the lack of respite support, the endless cycle of giving loving care without even the slightest break, the loss of friends who faded into the background when they had to continually refuse invitations, the need to stop working, and the high level of abusive blackmail (e.g., "If you go out, I could be dead when you get back") that shrouded their lives in guilt. They often experienced this blackmail even if they simply popped out of the house to purchase necessities. Following this conference, a small pilot project, supported by the Community Education Department, was initiated. It offered six different learning opportunities, for two hours each week, to give caregivers a break from the relentlessness of their roles.

The courses were based in the center and ranged from watercolor painting to gentle exercises. Caregivers came from the south side of Edinburgh and were most appreciative. They gave helpful information about the duration, location, timing, and emotional value of what they had experienced. Armed with the responses to the pilot project and additional information gained from the 3Ms Social Needs Survey, funding was sought and received to provide a range of courses to caregivers at convenient locations and at times suitable to them.

With great wisdom, the trustees of the center again delegated responsibility for the project's development and staffing to a subcommittee including health, education, and social service professionals, as well as caregivers. This formula had worked well before and would be an invaluable source of expertise and support as the service developed. The name, shortened to Ca(I)re, highlighted the fact that individual caregivers would be central to all the services offered to support them. It took some time for professionals to accept that short breaks, when the mind is occupied with a personal interest or learning experience, were as valuable as a two-week respite break once every couple of years or never, as was typically the case.

The following two years allowed for some degree of experimentation. It was interesting that many of the course instructors went out of their way to be extra helpful, because they themselves had experienced caregiving. The creativity of the caregivers in their evaluations also helped to drive the quality of courses. They often suggested new courses that would be helpful to them. A Balancing Needs course was developed and offered by a counseling service. Adult Basic Literacy and Numeracy courses were offered and supplemented by more advanced courses. Visits to art galleries were organized, as were visits to theaters to gain an understanding of backstage operations. A book club attracted caregivers, who, when funding was no longer available, self-funded it for many years. Gardening and cooking were well-loved courses and addressed different topics within those disciplines. Hill walking and writing skills were merged. Caregivers learned from park rangers, who took them on guided walks on one week. The following week, caregivers wrote poetry or prose about their experiences on the hills.

In due course, caregivers from the north of the city demanded access to the service. We were able to meet their request when an additional three years of funding became available. This new development meant we could take courses into the areas where caregivers lived.

Caregivers were invited to a one-day event in their local area when they could meet instructors of all the courses being offered and select the ones they would like to attend.

Many caregivers spoke of the benefits they received from attending events and courses. For some, the program was confidence building. Some made new friendships. As circumstances changed, some caregivers went on to further education or took on voluntary roles. All proclaimed the benefit of these short respite breaks, which provided social care, health information, and access to cultural activities and well-being in the context of life-long learning. As a result of caregivers' input, Ca(I)re successfully sought additional funding to create a bespoke befriending service for caregivers.

HEARTBEAT

The Eric Liddell Centre, now appropriately named the Eric Liddell Community, is the work of many hearts and many hands, local people who have reached out to their community with care and compassion. Their care and compassion reflect the objectives of the 1878 builders who also believed and lived by the Scripture "Truly I tell you, whatever you did for one of the least of these my brothers and sisters of mine, you did for me" (Matt 25:40 NIV).

Many thousands of people have passed through the center's doors. They have received a range of supports from loving hands that continue to reach out under the watchful eyes of those saints through whom the light flows. The center has provided support services for many trainings, conferences, family events, dance or exercise classes, and judo or tae kwon do lessons, to name but a few. A range of charities that have outgrown their offices and churches have based their evangelical efforts there.

Yes, it can be noisy. But if you listen carefully through the clatter of cups, the hiss of the coffee machine, babies crying, telephones ringing, singing, or dance music, you will hear the heartbeat of God as he continues to reach out through the care and compassion of this amazing community that carries out his work of honoring the man who honored him.

Bob Rendall
CEO (retired)
November 2022

Appendix E
Cognitive Dynamics

THE COGNITIVE DYNAMICS FOUNDATION (www.cognitivedynamics.org) is a 501(c)(3) nonprofit based in Tuscaloosa, Alabama, that was founded in 2010 in memory of Lester E. Potts Jr., a rural Alabama sawmiller who discovered latent artistic talent in the throes of Alzheimer's disease. The mission of the organization is to improve the quality of life of persons with cognitive disorders (such as Alzheimer's disease) and their care partners through education, research, and support of innovative care models that promote human dignity, especially those employing the expressive arts and storytelling. Current board of directors membership includes Daniel C. Potts, Angel Duncan, Lavanda Wagenheim, Gaines Brake, Don Wendorf, and Lynda Everman.

The foundation's primary program is Bringing Art to Life (BATL). BATL is an intergenerational service-learning program of art therapy, education, engagement, empathy building, and narrative. Offered to undergraduates at the University of Alabama, Birmingham-Southern College, and Loyola University, the course has been expanded for both high school students in Chicago and Rush University medical students. Students are educated in the neuroscience, clinical features, and impact of Alzheimer's disease and other dementias; the theory and practice of art therapy and other expressive arts therapies; mindfulness; person-centered care; methods of communication with persons living with dementia (PWD); life story/narrative; and perspectives on living with dementia, using both virtual reality modules and the lived experience of PWD. Students paired with PWD develop relationships while engaging in weekly art therapy sessions at adult day care, respite, or long-term care settings, under art therapists' and neurologists' supervision. A virtual art gallery experience in partnership with the Yale University Art Gallery is also offered. In art therapy, students elicit narrative material for legacy books containing art and students' written impressions, which are given to PWD/care partners at a final celebratory gala.

Appendix F
Finishing Well Ministries

FINISHING WELL MINISTRIES (FWM) is an important initiative that aims to change the retirement narrative. We believe and celebrate the truth that God wants to use aging followers of Christ to make a difference for him and to strengthen his work for future generations. FWM aims to encourage retired Christians and Christians thinking about retirement to fulfill God's plan and purposes for their aging years.

Culturally speaking, retirement means one stops working at a certain age. This new season often means embracing a more leisurely pace of life, personal pleasures, and then wondering what our new purpose in life may be. In addition, we are often marginalized by our culture, even in our churches. So we wonder . . .

- Why did God create our aging years, and does he care about this season of life?
- What are his purpose and mission for this season of life?

We believe God still has a compelling mission for us, and the Scriptures give clear guidance. In the Bible we discover that God's plans and purposes for us do not change with retirement. Consider the apostle Paul's encouragement for this season of life:

> For we are His workmanship, created in Christ Jesus for good works, which God prepared beforehand so that we would walk in them. (Eph 2:10 NASB 2020)

What are his "workmanship" and "works" he has prepared for us during these retirement years? His call is to keep growing, to keep being conformed to his image, to keep building his church, to keep being his ambassadors, to keep using our giftedness and our experiences, to keep being filled with the Spirit, and to keep on making disciples.

Then, in the not-too-far-distant-future, we will contemplate the words of the apostle Paul in 2 Tim 4:7–8:

> I have fought the good fight, I have finished the course, I have kept the faith; in the future there is laid up for me the crown of righteousness, which the Lord, the righteous Judge, will award to me on that day; and not only to me, but also to all who have loved His appearing. (NASB 1995)

Our years in this season of life are critically important to God and to us. FWM has developed resources to help. *Seven Essentials for Finishing Well* is a video/workbook series for personal growth or church. *What the Bible Says about Growing Older* is an insightful read filled with biblical insights about aging.[3] They are available on FWM's website or on Amazon.com. Podcasts and other resources are available on the FWM website (www.finishingwellministries.org).

Consider these words of the late Dr. J. I. Packer (1926–2020): "Runners in a distance race . . . always try to keep something in reserve for a final sprint. And my contention is that, so far as our bodily health allows, we should aim to be found running the last lap of the race of our Christian life, as we would say, flat out. The final sprint, so I urge, should be a sprint indeed."[4]

So we pray.

> So teach us to number our days,
> That we may present to You a heart of wisdom.
> (Ps 90:12 NASB 1995)
>
> Let the favor of the Lord our God be upon us;
> And confirm for us the work of our hands;
> Yes, confirm the work of our hands. (Ps 90:17 NASB 1995)

---

3. Habecker, *Seven Essentials*; Habecker, *What the Bible Says*.
4. Packer, *Finishing Our Course*, 21–22.

Appendix G
Spreading the Model of Dementia-Focused Respite Ministry

THE RESPITE FOR ALL FOUNDATION (RFA—https://respiteforall.org) guides churches in building communities of well-being and connection for people living with Alzheimer's disease and related dementias. These ministries are typically run by a one- or two-person staff and trained volunteers, with the church donating the space and paying the staff members' salaries the first year. Programs use research-proven interventions that:

- Enhance the quality of life for people living with dementia, by training volunteers to provide cognitively enriching activities and engage in meaningful interactions
- Improve the feeling of social connectedness among its volunteers
- Provide resources, support, and a much-needed break to the participants' caregivers

Because these programs use a social model of engagement, no medical training is required. From one to four days a week, participants engage in recreational and enrichment activities that fill their needs for relationship and interaction. At the same time, caregivers get a much-needed break as they leave their loved ones with trusted volunteers for four hours.

Attendees participate in interactive games in a friendly environment that supports independence. Enrichment activities include brain fitness (puzzles, word association, staff-led group questions, service projects), physical fitness (sport-related games, staff-led chair exercises), social (coffee time, lunch time), and creativity (arts and crafts, staff-led singing). Most importantly, participants engage in service projects appropriate for those living with dementia (e.g., packaging cat food for visitors to a food pantry). It takes friends and intentionality to make these service experiences happen, and that is why this volunteer ministry is critical in the lives of attendees.

Volunteers are often retired professionals who bring sensitivity, expertise, and personal commitment into an environment that is less like caregiving and more like a thriving recreational center. Furthermore, the cost to participants (approximately $40 a day from ten a.m. to two p.m.) is lower than the cost of in-home care, and scholarships are provided for those who can't afford the fee.

This ministry has several key features that make it easy to replicate and sustain, including no/low overhead, minimal number of paid staff, no medical staff, low tuition/fees to cover operational costs, and a large pool of volunteers who inspire donations from the community.

Daphne Johnston, whose background includes fifteen years as an executive director in senior living administration, began developing this model of care in 2012 when she established a volunteer-based respite ministry at First United Methodist Church in Montgomery, Alabama. By forging links with other faith-based communities to recruit and train volunteers, she realized the model could easily be replicated in other locations. As a result, in 2018, Johnston cofounded (with Warren Barrow) the Respite for All Foundation to expand this low-cost, high-engagement model of community care for people with dementia.

Winner of the 2021 Anne and Irving Brodsky Innovation Grant from the Alzheimer's Foundation of America, RFA has inspired twenty-five new sites that have served at least twelve hundred people living with dementia, as well as at least twelve hundred caregivers. Johnston's original respite ministry logged over one hundred thousand volunteer hours in ten years' time.

Appendix H
Grandparents Matter: Supporting Grandparenting[5]

THE NATIONAL ASSOCIATION FOR Grandparenting (NAFG—https://grandkidsmatter.org) is a nonprofit organization whose mission is to validate and encourage grandparents to leave meaningful and positive legacies for future generations.

Regrettably, a grandparent's influence in the family has often been overlooked and understated. Research demonstrates that grandchildren thrive when grandparents are proactive in supporting and developing relationships with their grandchildren, and grandparents thrive when they are actively involved in their grandchildren's lives. Further, when grandparents help perpetuate their values and a strong work ethic with grandchildren, the success of those they influence increases significantly.

NAFG conducts research and provides training, resources, and conferences to equip grandparents as they fulfill their strategic roles within the family. More than 75 million grandparents live in North America. Grandparents, with their extended life spans, challenge us to tap into and leverage this underused resource to strengthen families.

Over 1.4 million adults become new grandparents each year. In addition, many seniors who do not have natural children are grandparent figures for nieces, nephews, and other younger family members—as well as for neighbors and others in their communities.

---

5. Statistics and resources compiled by Ken R. Canfield, Grandkids Matter, Sept. 1, 2023.

Most grandparents achieve their status in their fifties. However, 37 percent of American adults become grandparents in their forties, with the average age of a new grandparent being forty-seven. Currently 60 percent of baby boomers are grandparents.

There is an acute need to provide support and easily accessible resources for grandparents (over 2.5 million) who are raising their grandchildren (over 7.5 million under the age of eighteen). Further, in the US, over 7 million households currently include a grandparent, up from 5 million in 2000.

Research shows that 54 percent of grandparents live close to their grandchildren (within twenty-five miles), and 46 percent wish they could live closer. Nearly three fourths of grandparents believe being a grandparent is the single most important role in their life and provides them the most satisfaction; 65 percent say they are doing a better job in caring for their grandchildren than they did their own children; and 70 percent believe that being an involved grandparent brings them closer to their adult children. Nearly all (90 percent) find great satisfaction in talking about their grandchildren.

Grandparents are lavish in their spending on behalf of their grandchildren. They spend $60 billion every year on their grandkids alone and invest $32 billion in education-related costs. Nearly two-thirds (62 percent) of grandparents say they provided financial support to their adult children and grandchildren in the last twelve months for items that include mortgages, education, day care, health care, and day-to-day expenses. Grandparents support communities as well. Nearly half of the nation's giving to nonprofits comes from grandparents. They also account for 42 percent of all consumer spending on gifts. It is estimated that grandparents control 68 percent of American's wealth.

In short, grandparents matter! They play strategic roles in helping families flourish, and NAFG was created to support their role as legacy leaders within their families.

Appendix I
Faith in Older People

FAITH IN OLDER PEOPLE (FiOP—https://www.faithinolderpeople.org.uk) is an organization based in Edinburgh, Scotland, whose aim is to educate, encourage, and support volunteers, health and social care workers, members of faith communities, and other agencies to increase their understanding of spiritual care and issues around aging.

Approximately 17 percent of Scots are sixty-five years old or older, and FiOP is a resource for the 3,700 congregations in the nation and for all people interested in providing spiritual care to the aged. Its work is organized around three basic themes:

- Dementia care and faith communities
- Mental health, older people, and faith communities
- Spiritual care education

The organization provides learning resources available on its website and through online and in-person workshops that help faith communities, health and social service agencies, and individual family members and friends respond faithfully and knowledgeably to the spiritual needs of older adults.

Its Anna Chaplaincy program aims to identify and train Anna Chaplains to serve all large- and medium-sized communities to help older adults "who feel isolated navigate the choppy waters of old age."[6] Since 2014 they have built a national network of two hundred plus chaplains trained in spiritual care. They serve people of all faiths and none, in residential care

---

6. Debbie Thrower, quoted in Faith in Older People, "Anna Chaplaincy," para. 6.

and private homes. The range of support is wide, from "just talking" to being advocates for those who are alone or feel disempowered. Their greatest impact is to help people feel "loved and cared about."

In 2020–21, FiOP completed a national research project whose aim was to identify and better understand the contribution made by older people in faith communities to volunteering, community well-being, and citizenship, highlighting the voluntary ministry that lies at the heart of Christian faith and is also echoed in all other faiths. This report is now helping to guide policy of both FiOP and the Scottish government concerning older adults.

Appendix J
Tuscaloosa Senior Ministry Projects

AGE-FRIENDLY RESOURCE DIRECTORY PROJECT

To understand and improve age-friendly communication between religious congregations and local (state and international) agencies, a local senior ministry association represented by local church leaders and an interdisciplinary team of gerontologists, practitioners, and college students initiated a six-part project consisting of two phases, using a "town and gown" community engagement model.[7] This initiative was aimed at (1) identifying current levels of service to older persons, the level of partnership between congregations and agencies, and plans for future senior program development; and (2) fostering greater access, communication, and collaboration between community agencies, congregations, and resources in aging using the internet. In phase 1, twenty-one local leaders from senior service agencies and ten local pastors were interviewed by two groups of volunteers and graduate students. Four other groups of graduate students and volunteers developed and distributed directories containing local, state, and international resources on aging to participating congregations and agencies. In phase 2, volunteers and students completed a larger telephone survey of approximately 16 percent of available congregations in the city to assess services offered to older persons. That survey also helped to update a citywide congregational directory, which was used to connect participating local congregations and agencies via the internet with the resources developed during phase 1. Practical problems involved in using the internet are discussed (e.g., limited internet access by underserved congregations), important service gaps are detailed (e.g., absence of disaster planning), and

7. Parker et al., "Helping to Create."

other outcomes related to future age-friendly work in the community are described.

For more information contact the James Houston Center (www.jameshoustoncenter.com).

TUSCALOOSA SENIOR MINISTRY PROJECT: ELDER/PARENT CARE PROGRAM FOR ADULT CHILD CAREGIVERS (AGEREADY)

In another community-based, age-friendly effort, two Protestant churches in different communities evaluated the benefits of an age-friendly program aimed at improving the readiness of adult children to provide parent care.[8] The organizers viewed elder/parent care as a normal, developmental set of medical, legal-financial, social-familial, and spiritual tasks requiring proactive attention by adult children with the assistance of their church leaders and professionals. A feasibility study was conducted with two faith-based communities, one in Alabama and a second in Texas. After participants completed a parent care assessment covering four domains of caregiving, adult children were given evidence-based information on how to complete salient parent care tasks. Christian subject matter experts in social work, gerontology, elder law, geriatrics, and spirituality conducted the workshops gratuitously, given their commitment to Christian service and their desire to share the latest information about caregiving. At the Texas site, adult children and their aging parent/s attended the training together. Overall approval ratings at both sites were very high; however, at the Texas site where both adult child and aging parents attended, the participants/dyads reported enhanced parent-adult child communication and trust among the participants. Future interventions should consider including adult children and their parents in the training. Consultation and copies of the full study are available at www.jameshoustoncenter.com.

TUSCALOOSA SENIOR MINISTRY PROJECT: REGIONAL FAITH AND SUCCESSFUL AGING CONFERENCE

In this brief report we describe a community and faith-based conference with elderly persons and their adult children that involved religious,

---

8. Myers et al., "Feasibility Study."

medical, and academic communities and a local senior ministry association. Lifestyle changes and individual and corporate forms of spirituality were affirmed using an expanded Rowe and Kahn model of successful aging. Faculty representatives from a broad range of over twenty professional disciplines conducted a series of workshops at a university conference center, which was underwritten financially by thirty church groups. The conference was hosted by a multi-church group, and over five hundred older people attended for free. Lunch was provided. Post-conference surveys were conducted, and extremely favorable satisfaction rates across all groups and churches were reported. The African American religious community provided critical leadership in achieving excellent African American participation rates. The model used in planning this conference has the capacity to generate collaborations across denominational, racial, and class barriers, and has the potential of helping to unify racially separated, religious communities around the task of promoting successful aging.[9] At the conference age-friendly themes were promoted by all the speakers and conference organizers: seniors/elders are needed, and seniors should seek God's late-life purpose for their lives.

9. Parker et al., "Multidisciplinary Model."

Appendix K
Small Volunteer Ministries That Can Bless Older People

HERE WE GIVE EXAMPLES of women who do not see themselves as developing programs, but who simply make a difference in older people's lives by being helpful.

Our medium-sized church[10] does not have a formal program for seniors, but it does serve seniors in a number of ways.

1. Each year the church staff helps bring together a Sunday noon luncheon where the church's high school students serve a meal to older adults and eat with them at the lunch table. This way older adults and teens in the congregation get to know one another in a natural way. The young people often help seniors by mowing or raking their lawns. Teens also sing carols to seniors at Christmas.

2. We hold two regular Sunday morning Bible studies for older adults. A retired professor leads one at which older couples and singles are challenged, fed spiritually, and enjoy ongoing fellowship. Another class draws together older women, many of whom are single due to bereavement or divorce, or whose husbands are away in the military.

3. One older woman who recently moved to our city and joined our church was feeling lonely. She proposed a fellowship time for older women at a local restaurant. That initiative morphed into what is now called WOW (Women of the Word), a bimonthly fellowship where the women share about the Bible and their daily lives.

10. Grace Baptist Church, Manhattan, Kansas.

4. Men and women of our church have often led weekly Bible studies in local nursing homes. Two of our WOW women recently started a weekly sing at one of our local nursing care facilities. A man who was recovering from knee surgery drew in a recent widow to round up patients throughout the building and bring them to the chapel to sing. She smiles and touches each patient lovingly and gives each encouragement. A pianist accompanies the group as they simply go through the songbook page by page. Often music deeply touches those who appear to be depressed or disengaged from the world. The words of the hymns teach and encourage, and the sense of fellowship is warming.

5. Our pastor's wife leads our church's women's ministries. An annual overnight retreat usually features our older women sharing their stories, lives, and biblical teaching with younger women. The younger women often include local military women and international students from the community's university.

Books can help people prepare for their later years and are often a source of encouragement for older adults. Here are examples of books local women have recently published:

Teri Gasser, our pastor's wife, recently published a book for aging women called *Choose Now to Grow Grand, Not Old: 12 Women over Eighty Show Us How to Smile at the Future*. She explores her own grandmothers' lives and attitudes, as well as the characteristics of other older women she has observed. Lively insights and challenges scattered throughout the book are real, challenging, and refreshing. Reviewers have commented: "entertaining," "shows you how to finish well," and "helps you celebrate aging."

During COVID, Kay Bascom, a Bible study author, wove together some of her own life experiences in the context of the Jubilee pattern described in Lev 25.[11] These observances keep appearing in the culture of Israel throughout the Scriptures. The Jubilee lens reveals God's fascinating plan for renewing his people's lives. Kay says, "Celebrating your personal jubilees can be like dress rehearsals before the curtain on eternity rises."

These are local examples of easily organized, but valuable, ministries that deeply bless and encourage people at watershed or fragile times in their lives.

---

11. Bascom, *Jubilee Journey*.

Appendix L
Senior Ministry Associations

THE CONCEPT OF AN association or network of like-minded nonprofits, businesses, or individuals is not original. These associations exist in areas as diverse as real estate, medicine, and sports. There are very few such networks, however, in the arena of ministries to older adults.

The general population is aging, as is the average age of individual congregations. The need for more focused ministry for, by, and with older adults is growing. Congregations across the country are stepping up to the plate with a wide variety of creative ways to serve the aged population. In some areas of the nation, congregations with senior ministries are uniting to share ideas and resources across communities by developing senior ministry associations.

An effective senior ministry association links congregations, leaders, and their participants into a thriving organization that encourages innovation, sharing, and fellowship. Senior ministry associations provide a vehicle to share information about successes and lessons learned that can bring inspiration, variety, and vitality to member congregations and the individuals within them.

A deacon at a United Methodist church in Maryland extended her work with a senior ministry in her own church to establish Winter Grace Senior Ministries, Inc., an organization that serves multiple churches and older adults in her area (www.wintergrace.org). The mission statement of Winter Grace Senior Ministries is to "Empower and Enrich the Lives of Older Adults through Christian Initiatives, Connecting People, Ideas, and Resources."

APPENDIX L

Winter Grace provides members with an online directory that includes the churches, ministry leader contact information, and numerous resources. A virtual discussion board allows for the free flow of information in a timely manner. An extensive online library provides print and video resources on a wide variety of topics relevant to older adults and ministries to serve them. Online conferences renew the spirit and invigorate leaders when weariness in doing good seems to overwhelm. Virtual fifty plus resource fairs connect seniors and congregational leaders with resources for seniors in the community.

Bibliography

Achenbaum, W. A., et al. "Patterns of Alcohol Use and Abuse among Aging Civil War Veterans, 1865–1920." *Bulletin of the New York Academy of Medicine* 69 (1993) 69–85.

Ajrouch, Kristine J., et al. "Convoys of Social Relations in Cross-National Context." *Gerontologist* 58 (2018) 488–99. https:/doi.org/10.1093/geront/gnw204.

Antonucci, T. C., and H. Akiyama. "Convoys of Social Relations: Family and Friendships within a Life Span Context." In *Handbook of Aging and the Family*, edited by Rosemary Blieszner and Victoria Hilkevitch Bedford, 355–71. Westport, CT: Greenwood, 1995.

Aten, Jamie D. "Aging with Resilience." *Psychology Today*, Apr. 16, 2019. https://www.psychologytoday.com/us/blog/hope-resilience/201904/aging-resilience.

Augustine. *The Confessions of Saint Augustine*. Translated by E. B. Pusey. Vrindavan, Ind.: Classy, 2023.

Bascom, Kay. *Jubilee Journey: Hope from Now to Eternity*. N.p.: Olive, 2021.

Berkow, Robert, and Mark H. Beers, eds. *The Merck Manual of Geriatrics*. 3rd ed. Rahway, NJ: Merck, 2000.

Blackaby, Henry T., et al. *Experiencing God: Knowing and Doing the Will of God*. Rev. ed. Nashville: Lifeway, 2022.

Bonhoeffer, Dietrich. *Life Together: The Classic Exploration of Life in Community*. New York: HarperOne, 1954.

Briggman, Anthony. "Irenaeus: Creation and the Father's Two Hands." Henry Center, Apr. 19, 2017. https://henrycenter.tiu.edu/2017/04/irenaeus-creation-the-fathers-two-hands/.

Calvin, John. *The Institutes of the Christian Religion*. Translated by Henry Beveridge. Lexington, KY: Pacific, 2011.

Campisi, Lynn, et al. "Legal-Insurance-Financial Tasks Associated with Parent Care." *Geriatric Care Management* 13 (2003) 7–15. https://www.aginglifecare.org/common/Uploaded%20files/memberOnly/GCMJournal-winter03.pdf#.

Caughey, Ellen W. *Eric Liddell*. Heroes of the Faith. Uhrichsville, OH: Barbour, 2000.

Chambers, Oswald. "Quench Not the Spirit." Utmost, Aug. 13, 2024. https://utmost.org/classic/quench-not-the-spirit-classic/.

Chittister, J. D. *The Rule of Benedict: Insights for the Ages*. New York: Crossroad, 1992.

Chynoweth, G., et al. "The Binomial Expansion: Simplifying Evaluations." *Journal of Counseling and Development* 64 (1986) 28–33.

Clayton, Larry. "The Port Rail: We Forget the Past at Our Own Peril." *Tuscaloosa News*, Sept. 27, 2020. https://www.tuscaloosanews.com/story/opinion/columns/2020/09/27/painful-parts-history-should-remembered-not-forgotten/3509357001/.

Colten, Harvey R., and Bruce M. Altevogt, eds. "Extent and Health Consequences of Chronic Sleep Loss and Sleep Disorders." National Library of Medicine, 2006. Bookshelf ID: NBK19961. https://www.ncbi.nlm.nih.gov/books/NBK19961/.

Crosby, Fanny. "Blessed Assurance." Hymnary, 1873. https://hymnary.org/text/blessed_assurance_jesus_is_mine.

Crowther, Martha, et al. "Military Families: Spiritual and Emotional Well Being Tasks Associated with Elder Care." *Geriatric Care Management* 13 (2003) 15–21. https://www.aginglifecare.org/common/Uploaded%20files/memberOnly/GCMJournal-winter03.pdf#page=3.

———. "Rowe and Kahn's Model of Successful Aging Revisited: Positive Spirituality—the Forgotten Factor." *Gerontologist* 42 (2002) 613–20.

Elliot, Elisabeth. *A Chance to Die: The Life and Legacy of Amy Carmichael*. Grand Rapids: Revell, 2005.

Everman, Lynda, et al., eds. *Dementia-Friendly Worship: A Multifaith Handbook for Chaplains, Clergy, and Faith Communities.* London: Kingsley, 2019.

Fabry, Chris. *Saving Grayson: A Novel.* N.p.: Center Point Large Print, 2023.

Faith in Older People. "Anna Chaplaincy." Faith in Older People, n.d. https://www.faithinolderpeople.org.uk/our-work/anna-chaplaincy/.

Fogle, Brienna M., et al. "The National Health and Resilience in Veterans Study: A Narrative Review and Future Directions." *Frontiers in Psychiatry* 9 (2020). https://doi.org/10.3389/fpsyt.2020.538218.

Frankl, Viktor E. *Man's Search for Meaning: An Introduction to Logotherapy.* Part 1 translated by Ilse Lasch. 4th ed. Boston: Beacon, 1992.

Fuller, George F., et al. "Helping Military Families Establish a Medical Care Plan for an Elderly Parent." *Geriatric Care Management* 13 (2003) 22–28. https://www.aginglifecare.org/common/Uploaded%20files/memberOnly/GCMJournal-winter03.pdf.

Gasser, Teri. *Choose Now to Grow Grand, Not Old: 12 Women over Eighty Show Us How to Smile at the Future.* N.p.: Steeped in Truth, 2022.

Graham, Billy. "Finest Hour 116, Autumn 2002." International Churchill Society, May 30, 2013. https://winstonchurchill.org/publications/finest-hour/finest-hour-116/glimpses-billy-graham/.

———. *Where I Am: Heaven, Eternity, and Our Life Beyond.* Nashville: Thomas Nelson, 2015.

Groom, Winston. *The Allies: Roosevelt, Churchill, Stalin, and the Unlikely Alliance That Won World War II.* Washington, DC: National Geographic, 2020.

———. *Forrest Gump.* New York: Doubleday, 1986.

Guthrie, Nancy. *The Wisdom of God: Seeing Jesus in the Psalms and Wisdom Books.* Seeing Jesus in the Old Testament: A 10-Week Bible Study 4. Wheaton, IL: Crossway, 2012.

Habecker, Hal. *Seven Essentials for Finishing Well: Fulfilling God's Plan for Our Aging Years.* Plano, TX: Finishing Well Ministries, 2022.

———. *What the Bible Says about Growing Older: The Exciting Potential for This Season of Life.* Plano, TX: Finishing Well Ministries, 2019.

Hanks, Tom, and Steven Spielberg, creators. *Band of Brothers*. Based on *Band of Brothers*, by Stephen E. Ambrose. Season 1, episode 10, "Points." Aired Nov. 4, 2001, on HBO.

Harvard Health Publishing. "Advantages of Water-Based Exercise." Harvard Health Publishing, May 10, 2023. https://www.health.harvard.edu/healthbeat/advantages-of-water-based-exercise.

———. "Protect Your Brain with 'Good' Fat." Harvard Health Publishing, Sept. 1, 2012. https://www.health.harvard.edu/mind-and-mood/protect-your-brain-with-good-fat.

Harvard Health Publishing, Editors of, and Gad A. Marshall. *Alzheimer's Disease: A Guide to Diagnosis, Treatment, and Caregiving*. Special Health Report. Cambridge, MA: Harvard Health, 2021.

Hazelden Betty Ford Foundation. "The Serenity Prayer and Twelve Step Recovery: Finding the Balance between Acceptance and Change." Hazelden Betty Ford Foundation, Oct. 14, 2018. https://www.hazeldenbettyford.org/articles/the-serenity-prayer.

Health & Nutrition Letter. "Fat Choices Also Affect Your Brain." Health & Nutrition Letter, Nov. 15, 2013; updated Sept. 17, 2019. https://www.nutritionletter.tufts.edu/healthy-eating/fats/fat-choices-also-affect-your-brain/.

Hodges, Chris. *Prayer Guide*. Birmingham: Church of the Highlands, 2023. https://assets.highlands.io/21days/2023/pray-first-guide.pdf.

Houston, James M. *Joyful Exiles: Life in Christ on the Dangerous Edge of Things*. Downers Grove, IL: IVP, 2006.

Houston, James M., and Michael Parker. *A Vision for the Aging Church: Renewing Ministry for and by Seniors*. Wheaton, IL: IVP Academic, 2011.

Houston, James M., and Jens Zimmerman, eds. *Sources of the Christian Self: A Cultural History of Christian Identity*. Grand Rapids: Eerdmans, 2018.

Houston, J. M. *The Transforming Power of Prayer: Deepening Your Friendship with God*. Colorado Springs: Nav, 1996.

Hudson, Hugh, dir. *Chariots of Fire*. Los Angeles: 20th Century Fox, 1981.

Kane, Robert L., et al. *Essentials of Clinical Geriatrics*. 8th ed. New York: McGraw-Hill Education, 2018.

Klemmack, David L. "A Cluster Analysis Typology of Religiousness/Spirituality among Older Adults." *Research on Aging* 29 (2007) 163–83. https://doi.org/10.1177/0164027506296757.

Koenig, Harold J. "An 83-Year-Old Woman with Chronic Illness and Strong Religious Beliefs." *JAMA* 288 (2002) 487–93. DOI: 10.1001/jama.288.4.487.

Landry, Robert. *Live Long, Die Short: A Guide to Authentic Health and Successful Aging*. Austin: Greenleaf, 2014.

Larimore, Walter L., et al. "Should Clinicians Incorporate Positive Spirituality into Their Practices? What Does the Evidence Say?" *Annals of Behavioral Medicine* 24 (2002) 69–73.

Lawrence, Brother. *The Practice of the Presence of God*. New Kensington, PA: Whitaker, 1982.

Lewis, C. S. *The Chronicles of Narnia*. 7 vols. London: Bles [bks. 1–5], Bodley Head [bks 6–7], 1950–56.

———. *Mere Christianity*. London: Collins, 2017.

———. *The Quotable Lewis*. Edited by Wayne Martindale and Jerry Root. Wheaton, IL: Tyndale, 1989.

———. *The Weight of Glory*. London: Collins, 2013.

Loconte, Joe. *A Hobbit, a Wardrobe, and a Great War: How J. R. R. Tolkien and C. S. Lewis Rediscovered Faith, Friendship, and Heroism in the Cataclysm of 1914–1918*. Nashville: Nelson, 2017.

Manning, Brennan. *Reflections for Ragamuffins: Daily Devotions from the Writings of Brennan Manning*. New York: HarperCollins, 1998.

Martin, James A., and Michael Parker. "Understanding the Importance of Elder Care Preparations in the Context of 21st Century Military Service." *Geriatric Care Management* 13 (2003) 3–6. https://www.aginglifecare.org/common/Uploaded%20files/memberOnly/GCMJournal-winter03.pdf#page=3.

McCaskill, G., et al. "Fatalities and Old Age: Reported Deaths from the Tuscaloosa Tornado." Poster presentation, Rural Health Institute, Birmingham, Apr. 2012.

Monteverde, Alejandro, dir. *The Sound of Freedom*. Provo: Angel, 2023.

Moody, Dwight Lyman. *Prevailing Prayer: What Hinders It?* Chicago: Revell, 1884.

Moritz, Joshua. "Are Spiritual Experiences Just in Your Head?" John Templeton Foundation, Aug. 15, 2023. https://www.templeton.org/news/are-spiritual-experiences-just-in-your-head.

Myers, Dennis R., et al. "A Feasibility Study of a Parent Care Planning Model with Two Faith-Based Communities." *Journal of Religion, Spirituality and Aging* 17 (2004) 41–57. https://doi.org/10.1300/J496v17n01_03.

NBC News. "Meacham Calls Bush 41 the 'Last Great Soldier-Statesman.'" NBC News, Dec. 5, 2018. https://www.nbcnews.com/video/full-speech-jon-meacham-s-eulogy-for-former-president-george-h-w-bush-1389347395683.

Orman, Morton C. *Sleep Well Again: How to Fall Asleep Fast, Stay Asleep Longer, and Get Better Sleep Like You Did in the Past.* Sparks, MD: TRO, 2017.

Packer, J. I. *Finishing Our Course with Joy: Guidance from God for Engaging with our Aging.* Wheaton, IL: Crossway, 2014.

Park, Nan Sook, et al. "Religiousness and Longitudinal Trajectories in Elders' Functional Status." *Research on Aging* 30 (2008) 279–98. https://doi.org/10.1177/0164027507313001.

———. "Transportation Difficulty of Black and White Rural Older Adults." *Journal of Applied Gerontology* 29 (2010) 70–88. https://doi.org/10.1177/0733464809335597.

Parker, M., et al. "A Parent Care Assessment and Readiness Intervention Program." Unpublished manuscript, last modified September 1, 2023. Microsoft Word file.

———. "Religiosity and Mental Health in Southern, Community-Dwelling Older Adults." *Aging and Mental Health* 7 (2003) 390–97. https://doi.org/10.1080/1360786031000150667.

Parker, Michael. "Building Partnerships with African American and White Churches to Promote a Good Old Age for All." *Generations* (2008) 38–41. https://www.jstor.org/stable/26555580.

Parker, Michael, et al. "Authors' Response." *Annals of Behavioral Medicine* 25 (2003) 157–59.

———. "Parent Care and Religion: A Faith-Based Intervention Model for Caregiving Readiness of Congregational Members." *Journal of Family Ministry* 17 (2004) 51–69.

Parker, Michael W., and James A. Martin. "Caring for an Aging Parent Is a Military Family Affair." *Geriatric Care Management* 13 (2003) 2. https://www.aginglifecare.org/common/Uploaded%20files/memberOnly/GCMJournal-winter03.pdf#page=3.

Parker, Michael W., et al. "Helping to Create an Age-Friendly City: A Town and Gown Community Engagement Project." *Social Work and Christianity* 40 (2013) 422–45. https://www.researchgate.net/profile/Adria-Navarro/publication/262567839_Evolving_pastoral_care_A_congregants'_transportation_ministry/links/00b4953bdaa775d77b000000/Evolving-pastoral-care-A-congregants-transportation-ministry.pdf.

———. "Multidisciplinary Model of Health Promotion Incorporating Spirituality into a Successful Aging Intervention with African American and White Elderly." *Gerontologist* 42 (2002) 405–15.

———. "Soldier and Family Wellness across the Life Course: A Developmental Model of Successful Aging, Spirituality, and Health Promotion. Part I." *Military Medicine* 166 (2001) 485–89.

———. "Soldier and Family Wellness across the Life Course: A Developmental Model of Successful Aging, Spirituality and Health Promotion, Part II." *Military Medicine* 166 (2001) 561–70.

Parker, M. W. "Abortion and Its Alternatives." *Social Work and Christianity* 7 (1980) 339.

———. "A Life Course Perspective on the Importance of Story." *Social Work and Christianity* (2013). Further information unavailable.

Parker, M. W., and D. K. Winstead. "Patient Autonomy in Alcoholism Rehabilitation, Part I: Literature Review." *International Journal of Addictions* 14 (1979) 1015–22.

———. "Patient Autonomy in Alcoholism Rehabilitation, Part II: Program Evaluation." *International Journal of Addictions* 14 (1979) 1178–84.

Parker, M. W., et al. "Aging Successfully: The Example of Robert E. Lee." *Parameters* 24 (1995) 99–113.

———. "A Case for Computer Applications in Social Work." *Journal of Social Work Education* 2 (1987) 57–67.

———. "Eldercare, an Issue That's 'Come of Age' for Military Families." *Military Family Research Digest* 1 (1996) 5–10.

———. "Employed Women and Their Aging Family Convoys: A Life Course Model of Parent Care Assessment and Intervention." *Journal of Gerontological Social Work* 40 (2003) 101–22.

———. "Juvenile Court Discretion with Status Offenders: An Analysis of Factors of Influence in Alabama." *Psychology Review* 10 (1986) 73–99.

———. "A Life Space Approach to the Functional Assessment of the Elderly." *Journal of Gerontological Social Work* 35 (2002) 35–55.

———. "'Out of Sight' but Not 'Out of Mind': Parent Care Contact and Worry among Military Officers Who Live Long Distances from Parents." *Military Psychology* 14 (2002) 257–77.

———. "Targeting Drunk Drivers: A Military Intervention Program in Europe." *Journal of the US Army Medical Department* 12 (1993) 38–43.

Parker, Michael W., et al. "Age Readiness." *Social Work and Christianity*. Further information unavailable.

———. "Family Solidarity: Geographic Separation and Contact between Adult Children and Their Parents." *Gerontologist*. Further information unavailable.

Parker, Michael W., and David Albright, eds. "On Life Review." Special issue, *Aging and Mental Health* (2018–19). Further information unavailable.

Pew Forum on Religion and Public Life. *Religious Beliefs and Practices: Diverse and Politically Relevant*. U.S. Religious Landscape Survey. Pew Research Center, June 1, 2008. https://www.pewresearch.org/wp-content/uploads/sites/20/2008/06/report2-religious-landscape-study-full.pdf.

Powell, Alvin. "How Social Isolation, Loneliness Can Shorten Life." *Harvard Gazette*, Oct. 3, 2023. https://news.harvard.edu/gazette/story/2023/10/how-social-isolation-loneliness-can-shorten-your-life/.

Regent College. "About Us: 05/Mission and Values." Regent College, n.d. https://www.regent-college.edu/about-us/mission-and-values.

Reinhard, Susan C., et al. "Valuing the Invaluable 2023 Update: Strengthening Supports for Family Caregivers." AARP, Mar. 8, 2023. https://www.aarp.org/pri/topics/ltss/family-caregiving/valuing-the-invaluable-2015-update/.

Roff, L. L. "Long Distance Parental Caregivers' Experiences with Siblings: A Qualitative Study." *Qualitative Social Work* 6 (2007) 315–34. https://doi.org/10.1177/1473325007080404.

Roff, Lucinda Lee, and Michael W. Parker. "Spirituality and Alzheimer's Disease Care." *Alzheimer's Care Quarterly* 4 (2003) 267–70.

Roff, Lucinda Lee, et al. "Depression and Religiosity in African American and White Community Dwelling Older Adults." *Journal of Human Behavior and the Social Environment* 10 (2005) 175–211. https://doi.org/10.1300/J137v10n01_04.

———. "Family-Social Tasks in Long Distance Caregiving with Military Families." *Geriatric Care Management* 13 (2003) 29–35. https://www.aginglifecare.org/common/Uploaded%20files/memberOnly/GCMJournal-winter03.pdf.

———. "Functional Limitations and Religious Service Attendance among African American and White Elders." *Health and Social Work* 31 (2006) 245–55. https://doi.org/10.1093/hsw/31.4.246.

———. "Religiosity, Smoking, Exercise and Obesity among Southern Community-Dwelling Older Adults." *Journal of Applied Gerontology* 24 (2005) 337–54. https://doi.org/10.1177/0733464805278132.

Rohr, Richard. "Time-Tested Wisdom." Center for Action and Contemplation, Nov. 19, 2017. Adapted from Richard Rohr, *Living the Eternal Now* (Albuquerque: Center for Action and Contemplation, 2005). https://cac.org/daily-meditations/time-tested-wisdom-2017-11-19/.

Ruder, Debra Bradley. "Circadian Rhythms and the Brain." Harvard Medical School, Summer 2018. https://hms.harvard.edu/news-events/publications-archive/brain/circadian-rhythms-brain.

Ryle, J. C. *Old Paths*. London: Hunt and Co., 1878.

Schaeffer, Katherine. "The Changing Face of America's Veteran Population." Pew Research Center, Nov. 8, 2023. https://www.pewresearch.org/fact-tank/2021/04/05/the-changing-face-of-americas-veteran-population/.

Simpson, Gaynell M., et al. "Support Groups for Alzheimer's Caregivers: Creating Our Own Space in Uncertain Times." *Social Work in Mental Health* 16 (2018) 303–20. https://doi.org/10.1080/15332985.2017.1395780.

Spiro, Avron, III, et al. "Long-Term Outcomes of Military Service in Aging and the Life Course: A Positive Re-Envisioning." *Gerontologist* 56 (2016) 5–13. https://doi.org/10.1093/geront/gnv093.

Stanton, Marietta, et al. "Reintegration Issues of Military Nurses: A Focus Group Approach." *Best Practices in Mental Health* 13 (2017) 1–19.

———. "Reintegration of Military Nurse Veterans." *Military Behavioral Health* 5 (2017) 163–71. https://doi.org/10.1080/21635781.2016.1272019.

Sun, Fei, et al. "Predicting the Trajectories of Depressive Symptoms among Southern Community-Dwelling Older Adults: The Role of Religiosity." *Aging and Mental Health* 16 (2012) 189–98. https://doi.org/10.1080/13607863.2011.602959.

———. "Predicting the Trajectories of Perceived Pain Intensity in Southern Community-Dwelling Older Adults: The Role of Religiousness." *Research on Aging* 35 (2013) 643–62. https://doi.org/10.1177/0164027512456402.

Swihart, Nancy L. *On Kitten Creek: Searching for the Sacred; A Memoir*. Greeley, CO: Cladach, 2017. Kindle.

Swords to Plowshares. "Quick Facts about the US Veteran Population." Swords to Plowshares, Jan. 27, 2021. https://www.swords-to-plowshares.org/toolbox-article/quick-facts-about-the-us-veteran-population.

Tada, Joni Eareckson. *When Is It Right to Die? A Comforting and Surprising Look at Death and Dying*. Grand Rapids: Zondervan, 2018.

Teresa of Avila. *A Life of Prayer*. Edited by James M. Houston. Classics of Faith and Devotion. Vancouver, Can.: Regent College Publishing, 2003.

———. *The Interior Castle*. Classics of Western Spirituality. New York: Paulist, 1979.

Tolkien, J. R. R. *The Adventures of Tom Bombadil*. London: HarperCollins, 2014.

———. *The Lord of the Rings*. 3 vols. London: Allen & Unwin, 1954–55.

Trent, John, et al. *The Blessing: Giving the Gift of Unconditional Love and Acceptance*. Rev. ed. Nashville: W, 2019.

Wallace, Randall, dir. *Secretariat*. Burbank, CA: Disney, 2010.

Winstead, D. K., and M. W. Parker. "Propoxyphene on Demand." *Archives of General Psychiatry* 34 (1977) 1463–68.

Wolgemuth, Nancy DeMoss, with Mindy Kroesche. "Betty Scott Stam: A Life of Surrender." Revive Our Hearts, Apr. 21, 2016. https://www.reviveourhearts.com/blog/betty-scott-stam-life-surrender/.

Wolgemuth, Robert. *Finish Line: Dispelling Fear, Finding Peace, and Preparing for the End of Your Life*. Grand Rapids: Zondervan, 2023.

Yancey, Philip. *Where the Light Fell: A Memoir*. New York: Convergent, 2021.

Zemeckis, Robert, dir. *Forrest Gump*. Los Angeles: Paramount, 1994.

Biographies

James M. Houston (MA, Edinburgh; DPhil, Oxford) is founding principal, former chancellor, and emeritus professor of spiritual theology at Regent College in Vancouver, British Columbia. He is the author of some forty books, including: *Joyful Exiles*; *Believe in the Creator*; *The Transforming Friendship*; *In Search of Happiness*; *The Heart's Desire*; *The Mentored Life*; and *A Vision for the Aging Church: Renewing Ministry for and by Seniors*.

Michael W. Parker Sr., LTCR, PhD, DSW, BCD (board certified diplomate), retired US Army lieutenant colonel, is the founding principal and the executive director of the James Houston Center for Faith and Successful Aging. He has active collaborations with interdisciplinary teams of faculty and directors of late-life ministries around the world. He is a professor emeritus from the University of Alabama and has held an appointment as adjunct professor with the University of Alabama at Birmingham, Division of Gerontology, Geriatrics, and Palliative Care, and currently serves as a research associate with the Duke Center on Spirituality, Theology and Health. He completed a postdoctoral fellowship in Gerontology at the University of Michigan funded by the National Institute on Aging. Dr. Parker has over ninety peer-reviewed, highly referenced, scientific articles on spirituality, aging, and caregiving. He served as co-PI and coinvestigator on the NIA-funded R01 UAB Study of Aging and was a John A. Hartford Foundation Geriatric Social Work Scholar (2001–3) and mentor and member of the selection panel (2011–13). He is coauthor with Dr. Houston on *A Vision for the Aging Church*.

Index

Abraham, as a man of prayer, 33
activities and decisions, praying before, 35
activities of daily living (ADLs), 11
Adult Basic Literacy course, for caregivers, 163
adult children
  encountering resistance from aging parents, 114
  of frail elderly as vulnerable, 121
  including with parents in training, 176
  lacking motivation for parent care training, 115
  preparing for parent care, 123
adult friendships, pursuing with adult children, 49
advance directives, 96, 130–31
advance planning, crucial for caregivers, 89–90
The Adventures of Tom Bombadil, most boring book ever, 83
aerobic activity, regular, 101
African American religious community, 177
age, dementia risk increasing with, 90
age readiness, Christ essential to, 7–8
aged population, congregations serving, 180
age-friendly programs, demonstrating the love of Christ, 150
age-friendly resource directory project, 175–76
ageism, 8n10, 62, 88
ageist culture, participating in, 8

AgeReady intervention program, 118–23
aging
  aspects of "successful," xvi
  basic themes of, xv
  excellent example of successful, 3
  of our population, 12
  prayer and, 34–35
  study on at the University of Michigan, 21
aging parents, 22, 110–23, 127
aging veterans, depending on caregivers, 153
aging-in-place facility, Mike's father in, 111
aging-in-place program, at Berry College, 34n2
agnosia (failure to recognize objects), 90
Alabama Department of Senior Services, 131
alcohol, avoiding, 103
The Allies (Groom), 68
Allman, Richard, 24
Alzheimer's disease
  assistance centers, 94
  as common, 90
  description of, 91
  as a devastating disease, 87
  Rita Houston diagnosed with, xvi
American Association of Christian Counselors, video series on aging, 4–5
amyloid plaque, dementia and, 87
animals, including in stories, 67

Anna Chaplaincy program, of FiOP, 173
Anne & Irving Brodsky Innovation Grant, 170
Anselm, on knowledge of ourselves, 28
answered prayer, biblical examples of, 33
anti-ageist movement, starting, 34
antique saw, symbolizing dementia, 93
aphasia (impaired speech), 90
apraxia (inability to perform motor functions), 90
Aristotle, on sleep, 80
Army Health Promotion Command, Mike turned down, 24
Army Medical Department, 21
art gallery, virtual experience, 165
the arts, beauty and healing from, 13–14
assessment, of possible dementia, 94
assessment process, of AgeReady, 119, 120
assisted living facility, life review group in, 65
Augustine of Hippo, 28, 46–47
AYO light therapy glasses, 82

baby, mother's face in focus when nursing, 137
balance related exercises, 83
Balancing Needs course, for caregivers, 163
Band of Brothers television series, 65–66
Barrow, Warren, 170
Bascom, Kay, 59, 179
Bascum families, 67
Baxter, Richard, 108
BeAgeReady.com, resources for care needs, 122
bedroom distractions, reducing, 83–84
bedtime routine, developing, 84
behavior problems, 97, 98
St. Benedict, on the divine presence, 51
beneficiary, of a trust, 128, 129
biblical reasons, for life review, 61–62
biological clock, affecting sleep, 81–82
birth, of Jesus split history in two, 14

blackmail, caregivers experiencing, 162
"Blessed Assurance" hymn, 72, 72n10
The Blessing (Trent, Smalley, and Stageberg), 23
blessing the next generation, 137–38
blue lights, avoiding before bed, 82
"boasting," on God's work in our lives, 62
Bonhoeffer, Dietrich, 30
book club, attracted caregivers, 163
books, helping people prepare for later years, 179
boy, crippled in bed writing Scripture texts, 108
brain, during sleep, 80, 82
brain health and mental fitness, global alliance for, 99–100
brain-derived neurotrophic factor (BDNF), 101
brain-healthy snacks, examples, 103
Brake, Gaines, 165
breakfast, as the heaviest meal of the day, 80
Bringing Art to Life (BATL) program, 165
Bush, George H. W., funeral of, 15

cabin on Yellow Creek, amazing stories about, 53–57
Ca(I)re, putting the I into care, 162–63
"call," experiencing, 73
Calvin, John, 47
canoe, pulled loose from its moorings, 56–57
care, for individuals with dementia, 96–98
Care Inspectorate, introduction of, 161
career changes, multiple high-risk, 15
caregiver support groups, 113
caregivers
  benefits from attending events and courses, 163
  feeling ashamed, 96
  help for, 98–99
  influence on a veteran's life and well-being, 153
  lack of respite support, 162

navigating nonessential information, 113
not prepared for the challenge, 7
playing the role of behavior detectives, 97
providing support to, 169
support for unpaid, 156
supported by Ca(I)re, 162
caregiving
affecting sleep, 80
delegating responsibilities and tasks, 132
journey with Mike Jr., 70
should not be a solo journey, 66
studies focused on interventions, 113
Carmelites, life of incessant prayer, 48
Carmichael, Amy, 36, 37
Caussaude, Jean Pierre de, 50
Center for Aging and Division of Gerontology, Geriatrics, and Palliative Care, at UAB, 24
Center for Faith and Successful Aging, in honor of James Houston, xvi
challenges, 10–11, 119
Chamberlain, Joshua, selected to receive the surrender of General Robert E. Lee, 41
Champ, Mike and Lane's dog (photo), 144
CHANGE Act, 96n14
chapels, praying in, 42
chaplains, national network of, 173–74
Chariots of Fire (movie), 57, 159
childhood, life review questions, 74–75
children
accepting and passing on a blessing to them, 137
damage from sexual abuse of, 49
getting closer to adult, 49
Jim's service to the Lord, 107
Children's Fresh Air Farm, influence of, 19
Chinese students, at Regent College, 17
choir programs, with caregivers and dementia sufferers singing together, 92

cholesterol, risk of Alzheimer's and, 103
Choose Now to Grow Grand, Not Old (Gasser), 179
Christ. *See also* Jesus
becoming closer to the throne room of, 48
as essential to age readiness, 7–8
as joyful, 58
presented himself as Savior, not Teacher, 14
relationship with, 7
Christian acts of love, 158
Christian life and identity, 48
Christian people. *See* senior saints
Christian prayer warriors, stories of, 41–42
Christians
being good wherever you are, 108–9
first meeting someone, 12
as the greatest storytellers, 72
needing purpose for their lives, 61
wanting to pray more, 35
chronic conditions, 124
chronic disease, affecting longevity, 8
church, medium-sized serving seniors, 178
Churchill, Winston, 71
cinematographers, at the University of Alabama, 65
circadian rhythms, 81
Claire (Jim's daughter), ministering as a flight attendant, 107
cleanup, sleep and, 82–83
clergy
facilitating a family meeting, 132
helping families cope, 99
reinforcing the importance of proactive parent care preparation, 115
cognitive and physical fitness, maximizing, 13
cognitive decline, 101
cognitive deficits, 89
Cognitive Dynamics foundation, 165–66
cognitive stimulation programs, 97
cold-water swim, preparing for, 56
communication, with God, 27

communion, with God, 30
community
　grandparents supporting, 172
　prayer and, 29–30
　prayer evoking, 27
　words of hope and kindness to, 30
community and faith-based conference, with elderly persons and adult children, 176–77
community times, with God, 30
comprehensive geriatric assessment, 125–26
Confessions (Augustine), exposed his former life, 28
congregational veterans program, 150
congregations
　having no idea how to age successfully, 151
　with limited resources forming partnerships, 121
consultations, by AgeReady local professionals, 120
convoy model, of social relations, 93
cooking course, for caregivers, 163
Cornelius, prayer of, 33
cortisol, disrupting sleep in older adults, 81–82
courses, providing to caregivers, 162
COVID-19, toll on the old and disabled, 9
creative arts, impact on individuals with dementia, 93
creative ideas, getting in sleep, 81
creative storytelling, 65–66, 68, 69
cultural Zeitgeist, current, 62

daily prayer, 35
Daniel, prayer of, 33
Darlington prep school, 23
DASH diet, 103
David, 29, 140
Davis, Charles, 13
day care experience, activities in, 161
daylight exposure, older people with limited, 81
de mens, meaning "out of mind," 89
Dean, Tony, 39–40
death, 14, 18, 45

dementia
　amyloid plaque and, 87
　caring for someone with, 88
　churches assisting caregivers of, 92
　defined, 89–91
　diagnosing, 94
　educating students about, 165
　exercise and, 101
　living with, 165
　nutrition and, 102–3
　obstructive sleep apnea and, 82
　people with separated from society, 86
　presenting major challenges, 101
　societal fear reaction to, 88
　specialist day care for people with, 161–62
　support for people living with, 156
　from a theological perspective, 92–93
　as the third leading cause of death in the US, 89
　those with died at a higher rate from COVID-19, 9
　types of, 90
depression, 52
Desert Storm, providing medical care for, 22
diagnosis, disclosing to a person with dementia, 94
diet, facts of, 103
discussion groups, on life review for veterans, 154
divine encounter, 54, 58
divine presence, 50
domains, representing challenges for older adults, 119
Donanemab (drug), slowing Alzheimer's, 95n14
double knowledge
　developing, 47–50
　of knowing God and knowing ourselves, 51
drug and alcohol consultant, to the Seventh Medical Command, 21
Duncan, Angel, 165
durable power of attorney, 129, 130

INDEX

Eareckson, Joni, ministry of, 109
early fathers, on the healing of souls, 141
early-stage dementia, determining the primary caregiver, 94
Edinburgh, Scotland, as a special place, 157
Edinburgh life review group, 64–65
Edwards, Jonathan, 46–47
Edwin Hawkins Singers, "Oh Happy Day" sung by, 57
elder caregiving, challenges of, 20
elder law attorney, parents consulting with, 127
eldercare training programs, evaluating, 4
elder/parent care, requiring attention by adult children, 176
elders' stories, moving from "casual" to "intimate," 72
Elijah, 33, 48
Elisha, 33
Elliot, Elisabeth, 7, 36, 37, 44
elliptical machines, 102
emotional woundedness, becoming aware of, 48
employers, aware of impact of parent care on productivity, 113
end of life care, actively planning for, 114
English Christian books, printing for publication in China, 109
enrichment activities, at RFA, 169
Eric Liddell Centre
  as a building for the community, 159–60
  change of name to, 158
  day care service, 161
  now named the Eric Liddell Community, 163–64
Eric Liddell Community
  short history of, 157–64
  of today, 155–56
Esau, 137
the eternal, recognizing, 12–13
Eternal "I Am," living in the presence of, 51

eternal marriage, as being "in Christ," 48
Eternal Physician, Jesus Christ as, 141
European Crisis Action team, 21
Everman, Lynda, 165
evidence-based guidelines, 116
executive function disturbances, 90
exercise, 83, 93, 101, 102
external cognitive aids, enhancing memory, 97
the extraordinary, discovering, 12–13
faith
  allowing God to develop our own, 46
  in older people, 173–74
  powerful effects of strong, vibrant, 5
  relationship with health, 116
Faith and Successful Aging, conferences on, 4
Faith in Older People (FiOP), 6n7, 58n8, 173–74
faith-based activities, involving dementia sufferers, 96
faith-based communities
  developing parent care training programs, 117
  disconnect with professional and academic organizations, 115
  insights from experiences of military families, 118
  planning for care of older members, 111–12
  programs and support services to caregivers, 116
  supporting aging veterans and their caregivers, 152
faith-based dementia respite program, Daphne Johnston's, 90–91
faith-based initiatives, in support of veterans, 152–54
faith-based interventions, 117, 153
faith-based organizations, 122, 150
faith-based parent care readiness and training, 112
faith-based systems, assisting elderly persons following disasters, 149–50

families
  assisting older individuals with mild dementia, 99
  Christ reuniting, 20
  life review questions about, 74
  as primary caregivers, 122
Family Caregiver Alliance, 130–31, 133
family caregivers, 101, 113, 151
family conflicts, reducing the likelihood of, 128
family consultation, by AgeReady local professionals, 120
family history, life review questions for, 75–76
family meeting, holding, 132, 133
family members, future messages and advice for younger, 135
family story, Mike's, 64
family values, transmission of, 135
family-social tasks, of AgeReady, 131–33
father
  child looking for acceptance and love from, 137
  Mike learning important things about his, 23
  modeled prayer for Jim, 30
  sexual molestation by a, 49–50
fifty plus resource fairs, connecting seniors and congregational leaders, 181
finances, arranging, 96
"finishing well"
  favorite movies about, 57
  opportunity of a life review to do, 65
Finishing Well Ministries (FWM), 57n6, 167–68
FiOP. *See* Faith in Older People (FiOP)
First United Methodist Church in Montgomery, Alabama, respite ministry at, 170
forgiveness, 19
Forrest Gump, Winston Groom author of, 68
foundation, Jesus as our, 14
Frankl, Victor, 36
Freud, Sigmund, 36
friends, life review questions about, 74

friendship
  God offering us, 29
  prayer as, 27–28, 46
fruitful life, nature of, 140
functional abilities, dementia impacting, 90, 95
functional status, 11, 95
funeral arrangements, instructions concerning, 140
FWM. *See* Finishing Well Ministries (FWM)

gardening course, for caregivers, 163
Gasser, Teri, book for aging women, 179
generation, declaring God's power to the next, 66
geriatric assessment task, 124–26
geriatric care, 124
geriatric care managers, 99, 132
Geriatric Fast Facts, on leading family meetings, 133
geriatric physicians, 10n13
geriatricians, on problems associated with late life, 10
geriatrics, distinguishing gerontology from, xvi
Gerontological Society of America, 24
gerontology, multidisciplinary fields of, xvi
global life expectancy, 8
God. *See also* heavenly Father
  allowing people to live longer, 36, 150
  being in the presence of, 16, 50–52
  choosing older people for missions, 10
  enjoying in late life, 9
  Eric Liddell sensing the pleasure of, 58
  Father, Son, and Holy Spirit transfiguring everything, 51
  forgiving sin because of Christ's crucifixion, 14
  goodness of, capturing stories of, 61
  led Mike into the field of aging, 24
  opening a door, 23
  prayer as friendship with, 27

providence of, 61
rescued Mike, 54
rested after creation, 81
sees and knows us, 28
using aging followers of Christ, 167
wanting a kingdom of priests and a holy nation, 107
watching over our needs during the night, 81
as with you wherever you go, 92
Gordon, Confederate Army General, 41
gospel, Edinburgh life review group aimed at sharing, 64–65
grace, 33, 140
Graham, Billy, met with Winston Churchill, 71
grandchildren, 135, 171
grandparents, supporting, 150, 171–72
GrandsMatter, supporting grandparents and great-grandparents, 150
grantor, creating a trust, 129
great-grandparents, as the new norm, 8
Groom, Winston, 68
growing older, 10–11, 12

Habecker, Hal, 57n6
hallucinations, in later-stage dementia, 97
hatred, for Jewish people, 11
healing encounters, with Christ, 71
Health and Aging Foundation, 126
health care, advance directives for, 130–31
health care crises of elderly family members, reacting to, 112–13
health care power of attorney, developing advance directives, 130
health care proxy, 96, 130
health fair, for older people and caregivers, 88
hearing aids, Alzheimer's and, 96n14
heart attitude, prayer as, 29
heart of wisdom, gaining, 67
heavenly Father, 54n2, 92. *See also* God
Heidi, Jim's youngest great grandchild, photo, 142
King Herod, 62

Hess, Bartlett, 102
hill walking, for caregivers, 163
history, learning from, 11
holiness, maturing in, 45–52
Holocaust, denying the historical accuracy of, 11
Holy Corner Christians, 158
Holy Corner Churches Centre, 158
Holy Corner crossroads, in Edinburgh, 157
Holy Spirit
  brought the word "wait" into Mike's mind, 56–57
  directing prayer time, 35
  guidance of, 36, 69
  voice of, 52, 58
hormones, production of, 81
house, built on the rock, 36
Houston, Christopher (Chris), son of Jim, xvii, 139n1
Houston, James (Jim)
  blessing his children and writing a letter to each grandchild, 138
  caregiving journey with his wife, 66, 88, 110
  celebrating his 101th birthday, 140
  on the eve of his hundredth birthday, 139–41
  journey to one hundred plus, 8
  photo with his children on his 100th birthday, 146
  photo with his youngest great grandchild, Heidi, 142
  photo with Mike in Vancouver in 2018, 145
  sleep habits of, 79, 80
  as a source of wisdom, xvii
  staying on track with God-given purposes, xvi
Houston, Rita (Jim's wife), xvi, 66, 88
Houston Center's military team, healing for veterans, 69
hugging, 138
human friendships, encouraging spiritual life, 29
humility, leading us to pray, 28
humor, 7, 81

Hurricane Katrina, triage system following, 150
Hussein, Saddam, 22
hymns, nursing home residents and, 179
hyperthermia, risk of, 56
hypothalamus, as the master clock in the brain, 81

IADLs (instrumental activities of daily living), 11
iatrogenesis, 9n11, 127
ideas, joy of learning and examining, 13
"image and likeness of God," people created in, 12
immortals, with whom we interact, 68
incarnation, mystery of, 51
independent living, evaluating capacity for, 11
instrumental activities of daily living (IADLs), 11
interactive games, RFA attendees participating in, 169
interactive health communications, 122
interdisciplinary medical care plan, benefits of, 126
intergenerational blessing, 138
intergenerational legacy, leaving, 60–76
The Interior Castle (Teresa of Ávila), 48
internet, practical problems involved in using, 175–76
interpersonal neurobiology, 93
InterVarsity conference, 16
intervention programs for caregivers, 113
interventions, 94–96, 98
Irenaeus, on God's divine presence, 50
Israeli Defense Forces, 11
Israelites, carried the tabernacle with them, 51

Jacob and Esau, story of, 137
James Houston Center for Faith and Successful Aging, 6, 24, 100, 149
Jeremiah, 7, 10
Jesus. *See also* Christ

on caring for parents, 110, 111
as the greatest example of prayer, 33
loved the outcasts and the marginalized, 71
obeying the words and examples of, 45
as our foundation, 14
Jewish people, systemic hatred for, 11
Jim. *See* Houston, James (Jim)
Job, 33, 55
John, Jesus entrusting the care of his mother to, 111
Johnston, Daphne, 92, 150, 170
Joint Commission on Accreditation of Healthcare Organizations, 116
joints of the body, less impact in water, 102
Joshua, 92
journey
  mapping out your own, 46–47
  value of those helping us on, 65
joy, prayer becoming, 28
Jubilee, God's plan for renewing his people's lives, 179

Kierkegaard, Soren, opened Houston's mind, 16
Kirkwood (aging-in-place facility), 20
Klemmack, Dr., kindness of, 41
klotho hormone, exercise increasing, 101
Knudsen, Far, led convoys of US ships, 68–69
Knudsen, Lane, power of prayer in a love story, 39–40
Knudsen, Olaf, Mike's father-in-law, 68, 69
Koenig, Harold, 5, 116

Lane. *See* Parker, Lane
Larson, Dave, 5, 116
last will and testament, updating, 127
late-Christian-life spirituality, aspects of, 19
late-life purpose, 109
Lawrence, Brother (monk), 50
Lee, Robert E., 41

INDEX

leg strength, correlated with cognitive function, 101
legacy, leaving an intergenerational, 60–76
legal documents, 127, 128
legal power of attorney, 130
legal-financial tasks, of AgeReady, 127–31
leprosy, 85–87
Leqembi (drug), 87n3
Letters from a Hospital Bed, by Jim Houston, 139n1
Lewis, C. S.
   characterizations of Jesus, 14
   on the immortals with whom we associate, 68
   Jim Houston's friend and colleague, 4
   Jim writing and thinking a bit like, 54
   kinds of Anglican, 108
   viewed every person as an eternal being, 12
   World War I shaped the writings of, 69
liar, molesting father as, 50
Library of Congress, on oral histories, 135
Liddell, Eric Henry, 36–37, 39, 57–58, 159
lies, living behind a wall of, 28
life, as a daily "dying" to the Lord Jesus, 45
life experiences, describing and discussing, 134
life over time, aging referring to, xv
life review
   biblical reasons for, 61–62
   creative storytelling and, 65–66
   groups, 63–65
   looking back using, 11
   sample questions to ask, 73–76
   sustaining an ongoing ministry, 65
   using to assess priorities, 62–63
life stories, 135
Life Together: The Classic Exploration of Faith in Community (Bonhoeffer), 30
life verses, examples of, 38
life-changing narrative, good memoir as, 67
lifeline to God, prayer as, 40
lifestyle, 10, 83, 91
light
   letting yours shine before men, 15
   maintaining circadian rhythms, 81
light supper, as better for older people, 80
light therapy glasses, 82
Lincoln, Abraham, 15
lives, working our entire, 10
living longer, 8–10
living will, 130
loneliness, affecting young and old, 86
"the long goodbye" disease, dementia as, 87
long-term care facilities, 34, 71
Lord's Prayer, 43, 47
lost sheep, parable of, 59
love of God, sharing unique narratives of, 71

Manasseh, cried out to God from captivity, 33
masks, people living with, 28
maturing, in holiness, 45–52
McClure, Dr., Mike's father's pastor, 19
McGee, Vernon, old "country" preacher, 6–7
medical tasks, in AgeReady, 124–27
Mediterranean diet, 103
megachurch, glimpse at prayer in, 35–36
melatonin, 81–82
memoir, writing a, 66–68
memories, keeping alive for years to come, 134
memory
   related to sleep quality, 82
   sharpening, 91
memory aids, mitigating forgetfulness, 96
memory albums and charts, 97
memory clinics, 94
memory loss, 91, 95
mentoring style, of Jim Houston, 4
The Merck Manual of Geriatrics, 126

Merton, Thomas, 10
middle-aged children, planning with aging parents, 131
mid-lifers, caring for aging parents, 110–11
Mike. *See* Parker, Michael (Mike)
Mike, Jr. *See* Parker, Mike, Jr.
Mike's father, memorial to, 19
mild cognitive impairment (mild memory impairment), 91
military families, 21, 42, 118
MIND diet, 103
ministries
　descriptions of promising, 150
　directed at veterans, 154
　embodying by the environment, 109
　fulfillment of, 13
　meeting genuine human needs of elders, 5–6
　with our children, grandchildren, and great-grandchildren, 68
　small volunteer blessing older people, 178–79
Minnie (golden retriever), 55, 55n3
miracles, place for, 53–59
model, of successful, resilient aging, 116–17
modern medicine, focusing on specific medical encounters, 124
Moody, Dwight L., on prayer, 32–33
"moral injury," traumatic memories resulting in, 70
mother and child, eye contact of, 137
multidisciplinary team, assessing dementia, 94
multi-infarct dementias, 90
Murthy, Vivek H., 86
myth, that older adults require less sleep, 83

Narnia tales, of Lewis, 69
National Academy of Elder Law Attorneys, 130
National Association for Grandparenting (NAFG), 171
National Institute on Aging, 83, 111, 131, 133

National Museum of African American History & Culture, on oral history, 135
National Sleep Foundation, 79
Navy wife, marital discord and, 49–50
neurological disorders, 90
neuroscience, of relationships, 93
nightly challenges, life circumstances affecting sleep, 80
"no gos, slow gos, or fast gos," older people as, 88
North Morningside Parish Church, selling of, 158
Nouwen, Henri, 14
numeracy course, for caregivers, 163
nursing homes, 88, 179
nutrition, dementia and, 102–3

obedience, prayer and, 27, 29
obesity, increasing risk of dementia, 91, 102
obstacles, in praying, 29
obstructive sleep apnea, risk of dementia and, 82
"Oh Happy Day," sung by the Edwin Hawkins Singers, 57
Olaf. *See* Knudsen, Olaf
Old Paths, J. C. Ryle's position in, 7
older adults. *See also* seniors
　capturing stories of, 134–35
　family meetings to discuss the care of, 132
　functional capabilities of, 124
　future messages and advice from, 135
　Sunday morning Bible studies for, 178
older Christians, 40, 61
older people. *See also* seniors
　death of, like burning down a library, 9, 23
　faith in, 173–74
　as a gift, not a burden, to the church, 151
　messages representing intergenerational transfers, 71
　not prepared for longer life, 7–8

requiring more time and effort to learn, 91
small volunteer ministries blessing, 178–79
oldest old, over eighty-five, 90
old-old (seventy-five to eighty-five) and oldest old (eighty-five plus) residents, interviewing, 65
olive oil, 103
Olympics, refusing to run in on the Sabbath, 37
Omega-3 fatty acids, as beneficial for the brain, 103
On Kitten Creek: Searching for the Sacred, A Memoir (Swihart), 66
O'Neill, Maureen, 58n8
online conferences, invigorating leaders, 181
online library, provided by Winter Grace, 181
optimal aging, xvi. *See also* successful aging
ora et labora, of medieval monks, 27
ordinary people, there are no, 68

Packer, J. I., 168
paideia model of education, 11
paideia-like learning experience, used at Oxford, 4
pain, causing agitated behaviors and problems, 97
parent care
  impact on adult children in midlife, 121
  improving readiness of adult children to provide, 176
  Mike's drive to create a program for, 111
  ministries addressing specific outcomes, 117
  officer satisfaction with having a plan, 114
  presenting a targeted intervention program for, 118
  review of relevant literature, 112–16
  severe stress associated with long-distance, 149
  significance of as a normal role, 122
  tasks involved in categorized into domains, 119
parent care planning, tasks associated with proactive, 115
Parent Care Readiness Assessment (PCRA) instrument, 118
Parent Care Readiness Intervention Program, communities of faith adapting, 119
parent care readiness program, 24, 149
Parent Care Readiness Program (PCRP), now AgeReady, 119
parents
  commandment to honor and care for, 8
  discussing future plans with children, 114
  involving in the training alongside adult children, 121
  loving children at their worst, 20
  relationship with affecting future relationships, 137
Parker, Lane, 32, 40, 70, 144
Parker, Michael (Mike)
  benefiting from friends, 93
  on expanding the military family care plan, 118
  experience as a caregiver, 92, 110
  family story of, 64
  friend's father cared for his elderly wife with Alzheimer's, 66
  photo of his family on his 75th birthday, 143
  photo with Jim in Vancouver in 2018, 145
  recommending the most boring book, 83
  stories of God's providence, favor, and purpose, 18–24, 54
  struggling with sleep, 79
  swimming, 101
  system of prayer, 37
Parker, Mike, Jr., 40–41, 70
Parker family, on Mike's 75th birthday (photo), 143
Paul. *See also* Saul of Tarsus
  describing fruits, 140
  on fighting the good fight, 168

(Paul continued)
   on the importance of parental caregiving, 111
   on love and appreciation of spiritual friends, 29
   prayed and sang in prison, 33
   on retirement, 167–68
   on serving the Lord, 108
people
   becoming more diverse as they age, 12
   as key to the success of any project, 161
personal answer, to prayer, 39–40
personal experiences, of prayer, 30–31
personal history, life review questions, 74–75
personal practices, of prayer, 36–37
personal prayer, as like one's fingerprint, 46
personal stories, how to tailor, 67
personality changes, in stages of dementia, 97
personhood, not lost to God, 31
persons living with dementia (PWD), communication with, 165
PET scans, limiting the number of, 95n14
Peter, 33, 50
Peterson, Eugene, 10
pharmacological treatment options, for dementia, 95
physiotherapist, working with Jim's tired and sore body, 31
place of respite, needing, 53–59
places
   of prayer, 32–44
   of rest, 53
plans and purposes of God, not changing with retirement, 167
plant-based diet, lower risk of dementia, 103
plasticity, of the brain, 93
positive correlation, between faith, religious attendance, and good health, 112
positive spirituality, defining, 116–17

postdoctoral fellowship, Spirit-led decisions to complete, 40
Potts, Daniel C., 165
Potts, Lester E., Jr., 93, 165
power of attorney, 127, 129, 130
power of God, to change lives, 20
praise and worship, value of, 42
prayer
   aging and, 34–35
   biblical examples of answered, 33
   community and, 29–30
   as the coping mechanism for caregivers, 99
   as essential, 31
   examples of, 43–44
   as friendship with Heavenly Father, 30
   as a heart attitude, 29
   inner, 51
   of Jesus, 33
   in a megachurch, 35–36
   for and with our children, 137
   personal answer to, 39–40
   personal experiences of, 30–31
   personal practices of, 36–37
   places of, 32–44
   tragedy and, 40–41
   as a window for the soul, 28–29
prayer breakfasts, as health-enhancing activities, 93
prayer closet, in military quarters or civilian housing, 42
prayer guide, giving alternative models of prayer, 35
prayer life, paralyzed by a father's faith, 46
prayer questions, Eric Liddell's daily, 39
prayer retreats, with students, 46
prayer warriors, 36, 41–42
"presence," becoming for others, 140
presence of God, 48, 50–52
pride, 69
priesthood of all believers, doctrine of, 107–8
priests, of God as a primitive practice, 107
primary caregiver, 132
primary degenerative dementia, 90

priorities, using life review to assess, 62–63
"prison ministry," Chinese publisher having, 109
processed foods, 103
prodigal returning home, 59
productivity, negative impact of parent care on, 113
profession, serving the Lord in your current, 109
professional and academic organizations, resistance to the value of spirituality, 115
professional callings, improving, 108
professionals, holding conferences, 151
programs, variety of new and well-established, 150
property, conveying to a trust, 129
prophets of Baal, failed in their prayers, 33
providence, of God, 67
Psalms, reading each day, 47
psychiatric symptoms, accompanying dementia, 90
psychiatrists, familiar with dementia treatment, 95
psychosocial outcomes, veterans experiencing, 153
purpose, late-life, 109
purpose-driven life, importance of, 61
PWD (persons living with dementia), communication with, 165

quality of life, enhancing for people living with dementia, 169
questions, creating a list of for older adults, 134
quiet place, waiting on the Lord in, 58
"quiet time," modeled after Christ, 35

races, having many to run, 58
ragamuffins, Jesus showed special affection for, 86
readiness assessment, 120
recumbent bikes, as good on the joints, 102
Regent College, 16–17, 108

relational wounds, that shaped us, 48–49
relationship, with God, 27, 46
relationships, neuroscience of, 93
religion, importance for many older adults, 98, 133–34
"religious and spiritual" variables, including in research, 5
religious communities, unifying racially separated, 177
religious leaders
  helping adult children and their parents, 117
  ill equipped to meet needs of older people, 111
  needing training and access to resources, 115
  preparing congregations for the unexpected, 122
remembrance, need for, 61
reminiscence and life review approaches, for older adults and their families, 134
reminiscence room, created to trigger memories, 161
Rendall, Bob, CEO of the Eric Liddell Centre, 58n8
research, opposition to spiritual variables, 5
research-proven interventions, programs using, 169
resiliency, 11, 53
Respite for All Foundation (RFA), 169, 170
respite ministry, model of dementia-focused, 169–70
respite programs, for dementia family caregivers, 98, 101
respite support, lack of, 162
rest and respite, embracing the restorative value of, 13
retirement, 10, 83, 167–68
Return of the Prodigal Son (Rembrandt), 42, 53
RFA. *See* Respite for All Foundation (RFA)
Rita. *See* Houston, Rita (Jim's wife)
roadblocks, starting with, 46

Index

Rocco (little dog), rescued by Minnie (golden retriever), 55n3
Roff, Dr., kindness of, 41
Rowe and Kahn (1998) theory, AgeReady program built upon, 123
Rowe and Kahn model, of successful aging, 177
Rutledge, Carrie, 40

Sabbath, refusing to run in the Olympics on, 37
sabbatical, taking from prayer, 46
safe room, going to, 53
saints, raising up an army of senior, xv
"salt and light," Christians functioning as, 14
Samson, 33
Saul of Tarsus, 16. *See also* Paul
Scriptures, 37, 47
Secretariat, winning the Triple Crown, 57
secular benefits, of life review, 63
sedentary behavior, negating benefits of exercise, 103
self-identity, dementia threatening the loss of, 92
self-knowledge, 28, 50
senior housing and programs, on college campuses, 34
senior ministry associations, 175, 180–81
senior saints. *See also* Christian people
  stories of, 65, 71
senior-ranking military members, risk for vocational, family, and health-related problems, 114
seniors. *See also* older adults; older people; senior saints
  with dementia participating in church, 92
  giving status in an ageist world, 72
  placed into nursing homes with COVID-19, 9
  relying on the internet, 122
  sleep tips for, 83–84
  young people helping, 178
seniors' home for assisted living, Jim's current ministry in, 107
Serenity Prayer, 43
Sermon on the Mount, 15, 36
service organizations, negative impact of parent care on productivity, 113
service projects, for those living with dementia, 170
service-learning program, intergenerational, 165
Seven Essentials for Finishing Well, video/workbook series, 168
sexual abuse of children, damage from, 49
shared memories, preservation of, 88–89
Sheen, Bishop, characterizations of Jesus, 14
Silas, prayed and sang in prison, 33
Simpson, David, 39, 40
sin, facing the realities of, 29
Sinise, Gary, as Lieutenant Dan in *Forrest Gump*, 68
sleep, importance for the health of aging bodies and brains, 79–84
sleep masks, blocking out unwanted light, 82
sleep medications, avoiding, 82
sleeplessness, undermining overall health, 81
small group life review, 64, 70, 72
smart home systems' IFTTT (if this, then that), 82
Smith, Colin, on Moody Radio, 13
Smithsonian Institution Archives, on oral history, 135
social and creative activities, for people with dementia, 93
social connectedness, improving among volunteers, 169
social isolation, 86, 96, 98
social media followers, securing rather quickly, 62
social needs survey, 160
social relations, convoy model of, 93
social workers, helping individuals with dementia, 96

societal changes, impacting families, 112
societies, age graded, xv
Socrates, death and, 14
soldiers, as prayer warriors, 41–42
solitude, Mike praying in, 36
"soul health," journey to, 141
souls, 14, 92
specialist day care, for people with dementia, 160, 161–62
spending, of grandparents on grandchildren, 172
Spirit. *See* Holy Spirit
spiritual aspects, of life, health, and aging, xvi
spiritual beliefs, experts sharing similar, 121
spiritual companions, spurring to love more deeply, 31
"spiritual father," Jim Houston as, xvii
spiritual history questions, asking in a life review, 73–74
spiritual-emotional tasks, of AgeReady, 133–36
spirituality
    importance of in successful aging, 116, 133–34
    neglect of by the research community, 116
    older people having higher degrees of, 34
spiritual-social domain, 136
sports, excitement of, 13
springing power of attorney, 129
stages, of aging, xv
Stam, Betty Scott, 44
Stams, prayer of, 44
Stephen, 33
stevia, as a safe sweetener, 103
stories
    on how God can work all together for good, 61
    of Tolkien, 69
storm, respite in, 53–59
storytelling, 62–63, 70
substances, discouraging sleep, 84
successful aging, 10–11, 116–17. *See also* optimal aging

sugar, as a contributor to Alzheimer's, 103
suicide, committing from depression, 51
Sunday morning Bible studies, for older adults, 178
Sunday School classes, as health-enhancing activities, 93
support strategies, for individuals with dementia and primary caregivers, 98
Swihart, Nancy, 66–67
swimming, as a heath-enhancing strategy, 101–2
symptoms or complaints, family member or caregiver compiling a list of, 125

Tada, Joni Eareckson, fought COVID-19, 9
telephone survey, updating a citywide congregational directory, 175
temptations, of our "worlds" becoming idols, 13
tentmaker, Paul as, 108
Teresa of Ávila, 47–48
theological perspective, viewing dementia from, 92–93
"a thorn in the flesh," Paul having, 108
3Ms Research Project (Marchmont, Merchiston, and Morningside wards), 160
3Ms Social Needs Survey, 162
Tolkien, J. R. R., 69, 83
Tolstoy, Leo, Christian faith of, 39
"town and gown" community engagement model, 175
tragedy, prayer and, 40–41
transformation, as evidence of Jesus's divine nature, 54
The Transforming Power of Prayer: Deepening Your Friendship with God, 46
translational research, sharing what we know, 151
trauma, 70, 153
Trent, John, 138
trustee, managing a trust, 129

INDEX

trusts, 129
Tuscaloosa senior ministry project, 175–77

unconditional love, 19
unforeseen events, preparing for, 122
unique ministry, capacity for no matter your age, 109
University of Alabama (UAB), mobility study, 5
University of Michigan, National Institute on Aging, 21
US Air War College, parent care readiness program, 24, 149
US military, research suggesting lack of preparedness for parent care, 114

vascular-related diseases, 90
veterans
 faith-based initiatives in support of, 152–54
 high suicide rates of, 69
 Vietnam War veterans, quotes from *Forrest Gump* enriching interviews with, 68
virtual discussion board, provided by Winter Grace, 181
A Vision for the Aging Church: Renewing Ministry for and by Seniors, xvi, 4, 65, 149
vocational calls, God's providence in Mike's, 20–22
volunteer ministries, blessing older people, 178–79
volunteers, at RFA, 170

Wagenheim, Lavanda, 165
Walter Reed Army Hospital, child and family fellowship at, 22
War and Peace (Tolstoy), 39
waste material, removed from brains during sleep, 79, 82
water aerobics, as a good exercise, 102
water of life, receiving to become fruitful, 47
"The Weight of Glory" sermon, by C. S. Lewis, 12n16

Wellspring ministry, 67
Wendorf, Don, 165
West Alabama Retired Officers Club, 34
What the Bible Says about Growing Older, 168
whole world, gaining, 13
Wiles, Jerry, 99–100
wills, 96, 128
window for the soul, prayer as, 28–29
Winter Grace Senior Ministries, Inc., 180–81
wisdom, xvii, 13, 14–15
witnesses, surrounded by a great cloud of, 57
woman, with the flow of blood, 71
women
 caring for aging relatives and for children, 121
 living on their own with lower pensions, 160
 making difference in older people's lives, 178
 ministries for, 179
working memory, decreasing when sleep deprived, 82
workshops, 120, 176, 177
world, gaining the whole, 13–14
World Health Organization (WHO), on aging, 8
World War I, Jim Houston's service during, xvii
World War II veterans, matching up with ROTC cadets, 34
worlds, identifying, 13
worship, 42, 92
woundedness, facing, 50
WOW (Women of the Word), 178, 179
writing, a memoir as one method of life review, 66
writing skills, for caregivers, 163

years, adding to your life and life to your years, 15
Yellow Creek, 55

Zoom, using, xvii, 150

www.ingramcontent.com/pod-product-compliance
Lightning Source LLC
Chambersburg PA
CBHW031812220426
43662CB00007B/615